C000100053

Published by 5M Enterprises Ltd.
PO Box 233
Sheffield
S35 0PB
United Kingdom

ISBN 0 9530150 1 7 © 5M Enterprises Ltd. May 1998

A CIP catalogue record for this book is available from the British Library.

IMPORTANT - PLEASE READ

The methods of treatment and control of conditions discussed in this book are guidelines only. Any recommendations given and so used are the responsibility of the producer, and the advice of his or her veterinarian should be sought in case of doubt. No responsibility is accepted by the authors or publishers for any application of the advice given in this book because each farm and region is different and responses cannot be predicted. Some trade names and their chemical compounds are used throughout. No endorsement is intended nor is any criticism implied of similar products not named.

5M Enterprises Ltd. would welcome your comments regarding this pocket guide. All feedback will be taken into account and hopefully help enhance subsequent editions.

Please write to us at:

5M Enterprises Ltd.
PO Box 233
Sheffield S35 0BP
United Kingdom

Alternatively e-mail us at 5m@fivementerprises.demon.co.uk
You can also contact us via our web page at:

http://www.fivementerprises.demon.co.uk/

and view other products that are under development or for sale.

PUBLISHED AND PRINTED IN GREAT BRITAIN

INTRODUCTION

Further to writing *Managing Pig Health and the Treatment of Disease* it became apparent that there was a need for a quick reference guide the farmer could actively use while actually working on the farm. This Pocket Guide is designed to do just that. To maximise its usefulness this guide should be used in conjunction with *Managing Pig Health and the Treatment of Disease.*

The guide is split into 4 sections, the first deals briefly with medicines and their use, the second and third looking specifically at pig diseases and the fourth on treating the sick pig.

The two sections on diseases make up most of the book. Section 2 looks at disease as it affects the breeding and sucking herd and section 3 looks at how disease affects the weaner, grower and finishing herd.

Both sections start with a table that highlights the symptoms a sick pig may show and what the likely causes may be. Details, including symptoms, recognition and treatment on the main causes are then covered later in the section.

The information provided is designed to help identify a disease problem and provide basic details as how this has arisen and could be treated.

Further background reading and discussion on prevention and control of diseases are covered in the main book *Managing Pig Health and the Treatment of Disease.* Other possible causes not covered in this guide are covered in more detail and depth in the main book also.

How to use this Book

IF IN ANY DOUBT CONSULT YOUR VETERINARIAN.

This pocket guide is designed to allow quick and easy reference to pig disease problems on the farm.

Sections 2 and 3 cover the diseases and problems that may be encountered by the pig farmer and each starts with a table detailing the clinical signs of disease (i.e. what you may see wrong with the pig or pigs), each with a list of possible causes.

The tables at the front of the sections 2 and 3 have clinical signs on the left and possible causes on the right. Items in **bold** indicate there is further reading in this guide. *Chapter/pp* numbers in italics indicate further reading in "*Managing Pig Health and the Treatment of Disease*".

Identify what appears to be wrong with the sick pig (use the table list as a guide) and note the most likely causes from the list on the right. Go to the causes in the guide and read about the disease. This will give symptoms, causes/contributing factors and list possible treatments.

The tables in section 2 are split into Sows, Lactating Sows and Piglets. If the condition is not in the Lactating Sow section refer to the Sow section as it will affect both.

It should be noted that a number of diseases/conditions are similar in all ages of pigs. In this case the disease/condition has not been duplicated and you are referred to the section where the relevant information is to be found.

To maximise the usefulness of this pocket guide it should be used in conjunction with *Managing Pig Health and the Treatment of Disease*.

REMEMBER
IF IN ANY DOUBT CONSULT YOUR VETERINARIAN.

CONTENTS

SECTION 2 - BREEDING AND SUCKING HERD

SECTION 3 - WEANER, GROWER & FINISHING HERD

SECTION 4 - MANAGING AND TREATING THE SICK PIG

1

Understanding and Using Medicines

SECTION 1

UNDERSTANDING AND USING MEDICINES

(See Chapter 4 for further information)

You are advised to consult your veterinarian when assessing information given in this chapter.

Legal Requirements

Medicines must be used safely and correctly in food producing animals to ensure there are no residues. Most countries across the world have strict controls over both the methods of prescribing and the uses of medicines.

Five groups

GSL: **G**eneral **S**ales **L**ist which includes a variety of medicines that are available to the general public over the counter.

P: Medicines that are available over the counter only from a qualified **P**harmacist where his expert advice and guidance can be given or supplied by a veterinarian for animals under his care.

PML: **P**harmacy **M**erchant **L**ists: Certified merchants who are able to sell from a prescribed list of drugs direct to the farming community.

POM: **P**rescription **O**nly **M**edicines only available on the direction of a veterinarian.

Controlled Drugs: This category covers the addictive drugs such as morphine, heroin and pethidine.

The major categories concerning the pig farmer are the P, PML and POMs.

When a medicine is supplied to the farm the following information should be available:-

- A description of the medicine.
- The date of manufacture.

- The date of dispensing.
- The date of expiry.
- The client's name and address.
- The species to be treated.
- The date of withdrawal.
- The dose rate and instructions for use.
- Name and address of the supplier.
- Manufacturer's batch No.
- The name and address of the veterinarian prescribing.

How Medicines are Prescribed

Most medicines have two names, one which describes the chemical which is the active principle, often referred to as the **generic name**, and the second, the manufacturer's own **trade name**.

Understanding Dosage Levels

All medicines have a recommended therapeutic range, expressed in milligrams per kilogram (mg/kg) of live body weight. This range is used by the veterinarian so that he can decide whether a higher or lower dose level is required.

For information:

1000ng (nanograms)	= 1ug (microgram) also mcg
1000ug	= 1mg (milligram)
1000mg	= 1g (gram)
1000g	= 1kg (kilogram)
1000kg	= 1T (tonne)
mg / kg = g / tonne	= ppm (parts per million)
mg / kg x 0.0001	= %
ppm x 0.0001	= %
1000ul (microlitres)	= 1cc (cubic centimetre) or 1ml (millilitre)
1000ml	= 1 litre

Controlling and Storing Medicines

Drugs that should be stored in the refrigerator 2-8°C (36-46°F)

- Iron injections.
- All vaccines including part opened bottles.
- Hormone injections, e.g. pituitary extract or milk letdown.
- Any bottles that have been opened and are in use.
- Any other medicines where the label indicates this temperature requirement.

Drugs that should be stored in a dark, cool place 18-22°C (64-71°F)

- Sedatives, vitamins and minerals.
- Stimulants.
- Antibiotics.
- In-feed and water soluble preparations.
- Disinfectants.
- Light and heat destroy drugs and freezing also has an adverse effect, particularly on vaccines.
- Provide a locked room or cupboard for all your drugs.
- Provide a refrigerator for vaccines and other drugs as required. Monitor the temperature daily.
- Agree with your veterinarian the minimum amounts that are required for a given period of time and follow his advice on usage.
- Make sure that all bottles are labelled for the correct use, that withdrawal periods are displayed and personnel are aware of them.
- Keep bottle tops clean, wipe with surgical spirit before use.
- Keep a daily record of all medicines used on the farm.
- Check regularly that medicines are in date .
- Dispose of empty bottles, needles and syringes safely.
- Make sure you have safety data sheets to hand.

Disposing of Medicines

This must be carried out with care to prevent environmental contamination and accidental human or animal contamination.

- Empty bottles should be placed into a plastic bag and disposed of in line with local authority guidelines or rules.
- Needles must always be removed from the syringe, and the syringes placed in polythene bags, marked "Syringes only" and incinerated.
- Needles and needle holders should be placed into a Sharps box, to be taken away for incineration.

Administering Medicines

There are 5 ways of administering medicines:

1. **By injection** - The injection can be either intravenous, subcutaneous, intradermal or intramuscular.
2. **Topical** - The medicine is applied to the surface of the body.
3. **Oral** - The medicine is administered through the mouth. Most injectable antibiotics are also available for oral administration.
4. **Via the Uterus** - Pessaries (small slow-melting tablets) placed into the uterus. Antibiotics can also be administered this way.
5. **Via the Rectum** - Not a normal method for administration in the pig, although in cases of meningitis associated with salt poisoning and water deprivation, water can be dripped into the rectum to correct the imbalance.

1. Administering Medicines by Injection

Injectable medicines contain the active principle suspended or dissolved in a liquid. The label on the bottle indicates the actual amount of drug usually as mg per ml. Each drug has a recommended dose level expressed in mg/kg or mg/lb of live weight and instructions as to its administration, frequency and any side effects or contraindications.

Example: Terramycin Q100 injectable solution contains 100 mg/ml of OTC. The therapeutic level is 10mg per kg live weight daily and thus the daily dose level becomes 1ml/10kg of body weight.

In practice, instead of referring to mg /kg, it is normal for the veterinarian to prescribe on the basis of 1ml/kg of live weight. Guidelines are usually printed on the label.

An understanding of the basic anatomy of the skin and its underlying structures is helpful if medicines are to be injected efficiently. See Diagram of the Skin. An injection directly into the skin or the dermis (intradermal) requires a tiny needle less than 5mm long. This is used by veterinarians when testing for tuberculosis. Fat has a poor blood supply and an injection into fat is poorly absorbed. Abscesses are also more likely to develop. Subcutaneous injections must only be given where there is a minimal amount of fat.

Key Things to Know

- On most pig farms 2ml, 10ml and 20ml syringes are required.
- Always use disposable needles and syringes.
- Use syringes with a side rather than a centre nozzle.
- Use only one drug in one syringe.
- Use one syringe for one injecting session and then dispose of it.
- Always wipe the bottle top clean with cotton wool and surgical spirit before use.
- Multi dose syringes must be kept in the refrigerator when not in use and cleaned and sterilised by boiling.
- Always keep part-used bottles in a refrigerator. Follow manufacturers instructions.
- Always use disposable needles that have a protective cap.
- Change the needle frequently and determine the frequency by the ease of penetration into the tissues.
- Always change the needle immediately if:
  - The end becomes burred.
  - You drop it on the floor.
  - It makes contact with the external environment.
- NEVER clean it with your fingers or wipe it with your clothing. Use fresh cotton wool and surgical spirit to clean the needle after 2 to 3 inoculations.
- Always use a separate needle for each individual animal when

injecting breeding stock to prevent spread of *Eperythrozoon suis* by blood inoculation.

Sites of Injection

The diagram Sites of injection shows the six main sites of injection:

- **Subcutaneous** - The ideal site for the small pig is inside the thigh beneath the fold of the skin or, beneath the skin behind the shoulder.
- **Intravenous** - There are three sites for injecting drugs directly into the blood stream, the ear veins, the jugular vein and the anterior vena cava or large vein that leaves the heart.
- **Intramuscular** - The common preferred site in weaners, growers, finishers and adults is up to 70mm behind the base of the ear. Small piglets are often injected into the ham of the hind leg because there is not much muscle on the neck. This is not recommended in growers/finishers because of the possibility of abscesses.
- **Intradermal** - This is only used by the veterinarian when testing for tuberculosis.

Self Inoculation - What to do

If you inoculate yourself accidentally you should take the following actions.

1. Report immediately to your manager. Ring your veterinary surgeon and/or your doctor.
2. Look at the label on the bottle. Does it give any emergency procedures?
3. Read the leaflet or data sheets which should be held on the farm.
4. If you are using an oil based vaccine (see the bottle label) go to the casualty department of a hospital immediately with the bottle. Such vaccines can cause blood vessels to go into spasm with potential loss of blood supply and consequent loss of tissue (e.g. a finger).

DIAGRAM OF THE SKIN

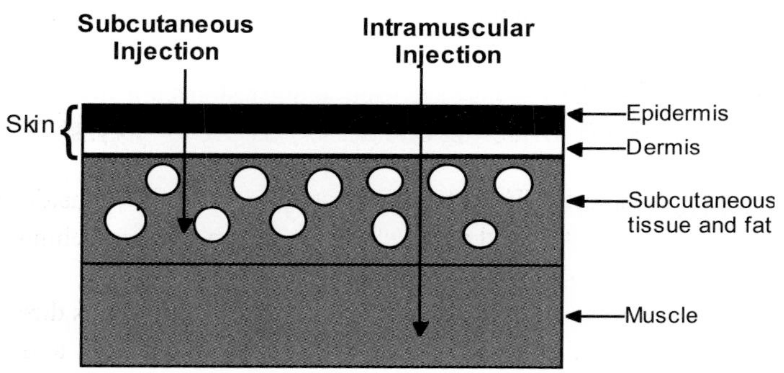

NEEDLE USE AND SIZE

Local anaesthetic	25 x 0.6mm (22g 1")
Iron injection	16 x 0.8mm (21g 5/8")
Hormone injection	40 x 1.1mm (20g 1 1/2")
Intra muscular	40 x 1.5mm (16g 1 1/2")
Subcutaneous or intramuscular	25 x 1.5mm (16g 1")
Jugular bleeding	50 x 1.5mm (16g 2")
Vena cava bleeding	125 x 1.7mm (14g 5")

SITES OF INJECTION

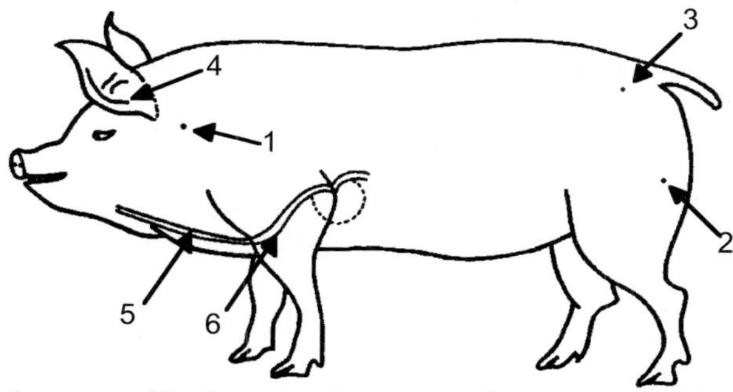

1	= Site for subcutaneous or intramuscular injection.
2 & 3	= Sites for intramuscular injection (piglets only).
4	= Site of ear vein for intravenous injection.
5	= Jugular vein.
6	= Site of anterior vena cava.

2. Administering Medicines Topically

These can be applied to the nose, mouth, ears, eyes, skin and feet. Treatments to the skin are either applied by spray, liquid or immersion of the pig and are used against skin parasites such as mange or lice or greasy pig disease.

3. Administering Medicines Orally

Water Medication

Treating pigs via the drinking water involves a daily intake of the active principle based on mg/kg of live weight. In practice however, it is better to consider this by the amount of active drug required per day per tonne of live weight of pig. Consideration should be given to wastage, possibly up to 20% with nipple drinkers. Examples of dose levels of water soluble drugs are shown in *fig 4-7 page 116* of the main book.

Water medication can be provided in a short period of time and be given easily and quickly in the early stages of disease. It also allows large numbers of animals to be treated at low cost, however it can also be wasteful in that it is inevitably given to healthy pigs that do not need it.

Key Things to Know

- Sick pigs often don't drink.
- The design of the pipe system may not be suitable.
- Water pipes tend to block up.
- Water tanks are small requiring regular administration.
- Up to 40% may be wasted due to inefficient nipple drinkers.

Applying antibiotic powder to water in header tanks

1. Calculate the total kg of liveweight to be medicated in tonnes.
2. Calculate the g of powder required for the 24 hour period. Add 10-20% extra if nipple drinkers are used.
3. **The water intake per tonne of liveweight per 24 hours will be approximately 100 litres .**
4. Calculate the total water used in 24 hours.

5. Divide the header tank capacity into the total water used which gives the times that the tank is emptied in 24 hours.
6. Divide the powder and add pro rata to the tank. Stir each time.

Example: Medication with Amoxycillin - 50% at 15mg/kg. Water bowls used. 4 tonnes of live weight at 30g powder per tonne = 120g. 400 litres of water consumed. If a 200 litre tank is available then 400/200 = the tank will empty twice in 24 hours. Place 60g or half the powder in the tank early in the morning and the other half at the end of the day.

Administrating Medicines In-Feed

The inclusion of antibiotics in-feed is the most common method of controlling and preventing diseases. In-feed medicines are prescribed by grams (g) of active or generic substance per tonne of feed. However, the manufacturer's product is normally available as a supplement - a mixture of the generic substance and usually a cereal base. For example Terramycin (OTC) 10% feed supplement means that OTC is present at a 10% level. Examples of in-feed medication are shown in *fig 4-9 page 117* of the main book. For technical and analytical reasons do not expect a 100% recovery rate if the feed is analysed. It can often be as little as 40-60%.

In-feed medication can be an effective means of control when used over several weeks however this can be wasteful in that it is inevitably given to healthy pigs that do not need it. In-feed supplements can also be used as top dressings, that is, sprinkling small amounts over the feed to administer the antibiotic. Top dressing is a very suitable method for small groups of pigs and individually fed animals, such as sows and boars but not for large groups due to the variability of intake of drug.

Key Things to Know

- Provide a separate bin for medicated feed. Bagged food is more expensive.
- The bin containing the medicated feed should be marked with the fill and empty dates to allow withdrawal times to be

calculated.

- If medicated feed is placed in a bin containing non medicated feed, the time and quantity of the medicated feed reaching the pigs will be unknown.
- There can be a delay in manufacturing and delivering medicated feed.
- Sick pigs often do not eat or have reduced feed intake and therefore may not receive sufficient antibiotic.
- Most in-feed drugs require a product licence for use in food producing animals and therefore the availability of drugs is narrow.
- Automatic feed lines make the application of in-feed medication to selective groups difficult.

Treating Individual Pigs By Injection

When you decide to treat pigs by injection (or orally) ask yourself the following questions:

- Should I consult my veterinarian?
- Have I identified every individual affected piglet?.
- Is this condition one that has been reliably diagnosed before or is it a new one?
- Is it necessary to treat it?
- Do I have drugs to treat this condition or are they readily available?
- Are there any welfare or nursing implications?
- Should the affected pig(s) be moved to a hospital pen?
- Is injection the best option or should I use a different method of administration?
- What dose should be given? Have I the right information on this?
- How often should the drug to be given and for how long?
- Are any adverse effects likely?

Then you should:

- Record when the treatment started and its progression.
- Assess the response on a day-by-day basis.
- If there is no response within 24 hours consult your veterinarian.

Other Types of Medicine for use on the Farm -

Sedatives

There are three drugs available for sedating pigs, acetylpromazine (ACP), azaperone (stresnil) and primidone (mysoline).

ACP (10mg/ml injection POM)

This drug is used in animals to prevent travel sickness and occasionally in pigs as a general sedative at a dose level of 0.1mg/kg liveweight. It is also useful for treating abdominal pain in cases of colic or to provide sedation together with local anaesthesia.

Azaperone (40mg/ml injection POM)

This is a sedative and analgesic widely used in pigs and is very effective.

The dose level is 0.5 to 2ml/20kg body weight. The effects of the drug are dose dependent. When used at 2ml/20kg the pig is completely sedated after 20 minutes and lies on its side. The lower level of 0.5ml/20kg will prevent fighting when pigs are mixed.

Some guidelines to dose levels of azaperone:

- Sedation prior to anaesthesia (1ml/10kg).
- Sedate prior to examining pigs feet (1ml/10kg).
- To prevent a gilt savaging her newborn piglets (1ml/10kg).
- To calm an excitable animal before farrowing (1ml/15kg).
- Prior to mixing or transportation to prevent fighting (0.5ml/20kg).
- To facilitate any manipulative procedure (1ml/20kg).

It is important not to disturb the pig for 15 minutes after injection. Distractions will reduce the effectiveness of the drug.

Primidone (250mg tablets POM)

This is an excellent yet little used drug for preventing the savaging of piglets particularly by gilts. One tablet per 12kg body weight per 24 hours divided into two doses given am and late pm is advised. Treatment should commence at least 24 hours before farrowing and continue for at least 24 hours after farrowing.

The tablets should be crushed onto the food. Consult your veterinarian.

Analgesics

Phenylbutazone

Some trade names:

- Tomanol POM injection.
- Equipalazone POM injection.
- Equipalazone POM powder.

This drug is very useful in treating painful conditions such as acute lameness and torn muscles, bush foot infections or acute mastitis. It can be given by injection, by powder or by mouth and its use will be advised by your veterinarian.

Vaccines

Examples of available pig vaccines are shown on *page 129* of the main book. Their availability varies from one country to another.

Hormones

These products are usually under the direct control of your veterinarian. As a general statement the use of hormones that act on the ovaries to stimulate oestrus should be avoided because the stage of the oestrus cycle cannot be accurately determined. However at specific times their use can be advantageous. Hormones used in the pig include the following:-

Prostaglandins

There are three uses:

1. Given within 36 hours post-farrowing to improve subsequent fertility and litter size.
2. To resolve endometritis or womb infection.
3. To synchronise farrowing by injecting the sow from day 113 of pregnancy. Farrowing usually commences within 24 hours.

Prostaglandins are potentially hazardous to women and should never be handled by them. Special provisions are required for on farm use. Consult your veterinarian.

Milk let down products

These are hormones produced by the anterior pituitary gland at the base of the brain. Their action is to release milk from the mammary gland and cause contractions of the uterus. They may be given to promote the farrowing process provided there are no mechanical obstructions. They are also useful in promoting milk flow when the udder is congested.

Hormones Used to Control the Oestrus Cycle

These can be used to synchronise oestrus in groups of gilts or in sows after weaning.

Regumate Porcine (POM)

This is an oil based product containing the active principle altrenogest - a progesterone substance. Given daily it suppresses oestrus in the non pregnant female. When removed the sow or gilt will come into heat.

Its main use is to synchronise oestrus by medicating batches of gilts daily for 18 days, (5mls per day per gilt is placed on the feed). At the end of this period following its withdrawal most gilts will be in heat within 5-7 days.

It can also be used in sows at weaning time to synchronise oestrus but this should not be necessary at a commercial level. Regumate should only be used in gilts that have shown oestrus. Some trials have shown an increase in litter size following its use.

PG600 (POM)

This product contains hormones that stimulate the production and release of follicles from the ovary. PG600 is used to stimulate gilts that have failed to show oestrus but in such cases it is not uncommon for only 50% to respond, and come into heat. Furthermore some gilts will be mated only to become pseudo pregnant and not farrow. It is better to cull anoestrus gilts - they are telling you they are infertile.

Gilts treated with PG600 should be served towards the end of the heat period.

PG600 can be used where there are anoestrus problems in first litter gilts. Litter size is often improved. Gilts are injected on the day of weaning and a normal oestrus follows. However if this is necessary, your management and or nutrition in lactation is probably wrong.

Electrolytes

When a pig looses fluids due to diarrhoea or vomiting for example it looses elements (electrolytes) such as sodium and potassium, and hydrogen ions. These must be replaced. A 15% loss of body fluids will cause death.

Rehydration by Mouth

This is the most practical method for use in sucking pigs and weaners. Glucose water and electrolytes when combined with the amino acid glycine are well absorbed from the small intestine.

A typical electrolyte formulation would comprise

	%
Glucose	67.5
Sodium chloride	14.3
Glycine	10.4
Potassium dihydrogen phosphate	6.8
Citric acid	0.8
Potassium citrate	0.2

It is mixed with water at a rate of 30g per litre for the first 24 hours and followed by 15g per litre until the pig has recovered. The solution should be provided fresh daily in easily accessible drinkers.

A number of commercial electrolyte solutions are available but all should contain glycine.

2

Recognising and Treating Diseases in the Breeding and Sucking Herd

SECTION 2

Recognising and Treating Diseases in the Breeding and Sucking Herd

Use the following table to identify the possible cause of disease based on your clinical observations:

Dry Sows

Clinical signs	Causes / contributing factors
Abdomen distended (Blown up)	Constipation Excess gas in large bowel Faulty nutrition *(Chapter 14)* Too much food **Torsion of stomach or intestines** *
Abnormal heat (oestrus)	Cystic ovaries * **Fungal poisoning**
Abortion *(See Chapters 5 & 6)*	**Brucellosis** Disease - generalised **Erysipelas** Incorrect lighting Lack of boar contact **Leptospirosis** Poor environment * Poor light Poor nutrition *(Chapter 14)* Porcine reproductive and respiratory syndrome (PRRS) Virus infections *(Chapter 6)*

Clinical signs	Causes / contributing factors
Abscesses	**Bursitis** **Bush foot** Faulty injections * **Fractures** Septicaemia Trauma **Vice - Abnormal behaviour**
Anaemia	**Eperythrozoonosis (Epe)** **Gastric ulcers** **Haematoma** Internal bleeding * Loss of blood visible **Porcine enteropathy (PE) - Bloody gut** **Prolapse of the rectum** **Torsion of the stomach and intestines**
Anoestrus (lack of heat)	Disease - generalised **Fungal poisoning** Lack of boar contact Low feed intake and/or poor nutrition. Low temperature and/or low light intensity **Metritis** - inflammation of the womb **Parasites** Specific diseases e.g. **PRRS, Mastitis** Stress * See also thin sows *(See Chapter 5)*
Arthritis	See **Lameness**
Blindness	**Botulism** Lead poisoning *(chapter 13)*

Clinical signs	Causes / contributing factors
(Cont.)	**Meningitis** **Salt poisoning (Water deprivation)** *
Blisters	**Foot and mouth disease (FMD)** (Sec.3) **Swine vesicular disease (SVD)** (Sec. 3) Other vesicular diseases *(Chapter 12)*
Blood from/on nose	Acute **pneumonia** **Atrophic rhinitis (AR) (PAR)** Cannibalism **Prolapse of the rectum** Ruptured blood vessel Trauma
Blood from the vulva or vagina	**Abortion** **Cystitis / pyelonephritis** Dead foetuses. **Haematoma**. Physical damage/injury Ruptured blood vessel in womb or vulva * Trauma to vulva *
Blood in faeces	**Gastric ulcers** * **Parasites** **Porcine enteropathy (PE) - Bloody gut** **Prolapse of the rectum** Ruptured blood vessel **Swine Dysentery (SD)** Trauma. Warfarin poisoning *(Chapter 13)*
Blood in semen	Ruptured blood vessel. Ulceration of urethra, **Mange** *

Clinical signs	Causes / contributing factors
Blood in urine	Acute **Cystitis / Pyelonephritis** **Leptospirosis**
Coughing (Unusual unless a new disease has entered the herd).	**Aujeszky's disease (AD) (PR)** * Dust **Enzootic pneumonia (EP)** Lung abscesses **Parasites** - Ascarids or lung worms **Pasteurellosis** (Section 3) **Pneumonia** **Porcine reproductive and respiratory syndrome (PRRS)** **Salmonellosis** **Swine fevers** **Swine influenza (SI)** * Toxic gases *(Chapter 13)*
Cuts and bruises	Fighting Trauma from the environment
Diamond shaped lesions	**Erysipelas**
Diarrhoea	**Colitis** (Section 3) Diet changes *, Over eating **Parasites** Poor nutrition *(Chapter 14)* **Porcine enteropathy (PE)** **- Bloody gut** (Gilts) **Porcine epidemic diarrhoea (PED)** * **Salmonellosis.** **Swine dysentery (SD)** **Swine fevers** **Transmissible gastro-enteritis (TGE)** *

Clinical signs	Causes / contributing factors
Discharge from eyes.	Blocked tear ducts Conjunctivitis Previous rhinitis damage Specific respiratory diseases *
Discharge from nose	**Atrophic rhinitis (AR) (PAR)** **Electrocution** Specific respiratory diseases Ruptured blood vessel Other acute specific diseases (uncommon) e.g. **App**
Discolouration of skin Reddening, Blueing (cyanosis)	Acute **Actinobacillus pleuropneumonia (App)** (Section 3) Dermatitis **Erysipelas** **Frost bite** **Pneumonia** Poor circulation **Porcine reproductive and respiratory syndrome (PRRS)** **Porcine stress syndrome (PSS)** **Salmonellosis** **Sunburn** * Toxic state
Dog sitting position	Fractured hip or long bones * Fractured spine * Muscle trauma Ruptured disc Spinal abscesses **Swine fevers** See also nervous symptoms

Clinical signs	Causes / contributing factors
Fever - increased temperature	**Erysipelas** **Mastitis** **Salmonellosis** Septicaemia Specific diseases e.g. **PRRS** * **Swine Influenza (SI)** *
Fits - convulsions	**Middle ear infections** **Salt poisoning (Water deprivation)** See also nervous signs
Fractures	**Electrocution** Fighting **Leg weakness, Osteochondrosis (OCD)** Nutritional inadequacies *(Chapter 14)* **Osteomalacia (OM)** Trauma * See also **Lameness**
Gangrene i.e. black smelling dead tissue	**Clostridial diseases** **Ergot poisoning** (See **fungal poisoning**) **Frost bite** **Mastitis** * Poisons - other *(Chapter 13)* **Salmonellosis** Septicaemias * Thrombosis
Greasy skin	Excess skin oils * Localised **greasy pig disease** **Mange** Pustular dermatitis *(Chapter 10)*

Clinical signs	Causes / contributing factors
Grinding teeth	Infection in mouth Kidney infection Pain (colic) * Tooth decay **Torsion of the stomach and intestines**
Haemorrhage	**Swine fevers** **Thrombocytopaenic purpura** See blood
Hairiness	Bad environment * Generalised disease / fever Low temperature Poor nutrition *
Head on one side or shaking	Brain abscess **Eclampsia** **Haematoma** of the ear **Mange** **Meningitis** **Middle ear infection** * **Porcine reproductive and respiratory syndrome (PRRS)** **Porcine stress syndrome (PSS)** **Salt poisoning (Water deprivation)**
Heavy breathing	**Agalactia** - No milk Excess heat **Fever** **Pneumonia** * Poisonings *(Chapter 13)* **Porcine stress syndrome (PSS)** **Swine influenza (SI)** *

Clinical signs	Causes / contributing factors
(Cont.)	Specific diseases i.e. Respiratory diseases
Incoordination	See **Lameness**
Infertility	**Abortions** **Aujeszky's disease (AD) (PR)** Boar failure **Erysipelas** **Fungal poisoning** **Leptospirosis** **Metritis** Other specific diseases **(See Chapter 5)* Poor management / environment * Poor nutrition *(Chapter 14)* **Porcine parvovirus (PPV)** **Porcine reproductive and respiratory syndrome (PRRS)** Sow failures - age - breed **Swine influenza (SI)** See also anoestrus
Inflamed skin	**Swine Pox** (Section 3) Pustular dermatitis *(Chapter 10)*
Jaundice (yellow skin)	**Anaemia** **Leptospirosis** * Liver failure Poisons *(Chapter 13)*
Jerky eye movements - Nystagmus	**Meningitis** * **Middle ear infection.** **Salt poisoning (Water deprivation)**

Clinical signs	Causes / contributing factors
Lameness	**Arthritis** **Back muscle necrosis** **Bursitis** **Bush foot / sand crack / foot rot**. * **Erysipelas** **Foot-and-mouth disease (FMD)** (Sec. 3) **Fractures** **Glässers disease** in gilts **Laminitis** (uncommon) **Leg weakness (OCD)** * Muscle tearing **Mycoplasma arthritis** in gilts Nutritional deficiencies *(Chapter 14)* **Osteomalacia (OM)** Poisoning *(Chapter 13)* **Porcine stress syndrome (PSS)** Spinal and/or pelvic damage. **Swine vesicular disease (SVD)** (Sec. 3) Torn muscle *
Loss of balance	See **Lameness**
Mastitis	**Abscesses** Infection in lactation or at weaning * Specific bacterial infections Trauma to teats
Mortality	**Actinobacillus pleuropneumonia (App)** (Section 3) Acute **cystitis / pyelonephritis** * **Clostridial disease** Dead foetuses **Electrocution**

Clinical signs	Causes / contributing factors
(Cont.)	**Erysipelas** Excess heat Fighting **Gastric ulcers** Haemorrhage Heart failure * **Metritis** Poisoning *(Chapter 13)* **Porcine enteropathy (PE)** **- Bloody gut** - gilts **Porcine stress syndrome (PSS)** Pregnancy catastrophes e.g. - torsion, haemorrhages **Prolapses** **Torsion of the stomach and intestines** *
Mucus/ pus in urine	**Cystitis / pyelonephritis**
Muscle trembling	**Eclampsia** **Fever** **Heat stroke** **Meningitis** Muscle tearing **Porcine stress syndrome (PSS**) * Rabies **Salt poisoning (Water deprivation**) **Tetanus** See also nervous symptoms
Navel bleeding	Mycotoxins *(Chapter 13)* Nutritional causes *(Chapter 14)* Poisoning *(Chapter 13)* Shavings or bedding

Clinical signs	Causes / contributing factors
(Cont.)	Trauma to navel cord Use of prostaglandins
Nervous symptoms (various)	Abscess in the brain or spine **Aujeszky's disease (AD) (PR)** **Glässers disease (Hps)** **Leg weakness, Osteochondrosis (OCD)** **Meningitis** **Middle ear infections** Poisoning *(Chapter 13)* **Rabies** **Salt poisoning (Water deprivation)** * Septicaemia **Swine fevers**
Not eating (Inappetence) Temperature normal	Constipation **Cystitis / pyelonephritis** * Dead foetuses * **Gastric ulcers** Indigestion * Nutritional problems *(Chapter 14)* Pain **Peritonitis** **Porcine reproductive and respiratory syndrome (PRRS)** **Salt poisoning (Water deprivation)** Sow failures Unpalatable food See also **Lameness**
Not eating (Inappetence) Temperature elevated	Acute **cystitis / pyelonephritis** Dead piglets inside the womb **Erysipelas** *

Clinical signs	Causes / contributing factors
(Cont.)	**Mastitis** * **Meningitis** **Metritis** (womb infection) **Pneumonia** **Porcine reproductive and respiratory syndrome (PRRS)** **Salmonellosis** Septicaemia (Blood infection) * **Swine influenza (SI)** * Torsion of the womb Water shortage See also **fever**
Pain	**Arthritis** **Back muscle necrosis** **Bush foot** Colic **Fractures** **Gastric ulcers** Muscle tearing * **Mycoplasma arthritis** **Peritonitis** **Torsion of the stomach and intestines**
Pale pigs	**Anaemia** **Eperythrozoonosis (Epe)** **Gastric ulcers** * Haemorrhage **Parasites** **Porcine enteropathy (PE) - Bloody gut**
Paralysis	**Botulism** Fractured spine

Clinical signs	**Causes / contributing factors**
(Cont.)	**Leg weakness, Osteochondrosis (OCD)** **Rabies,** See also nervous symptoms
Pimples and/or small bite marks	Fly bites **Mange** * Pustular dermatitis * *(Chapter 10)* Trauma
Pregnancy failure	Mating procedures *(Chapter 5)* Nutritional inadequacies *(Chapter 14)* Poor environment *(Chapter 5)* Poor management *(Chapter 5)*
Prolapse of bladder	A poor sphincter muscle Possibly **cystitis** The presence of calculi and continual straining Unknown factors
Prolapse of rectum	Excess gas in the bowel Increased abdominal pressure Nutritional factors *(Chapter 14)* Prolonged lying on a slope Rectal damage at mating Shortage of water
Prolapse of uterus (womb)	Faulty farrowing mechanisms Large litters Old sows Previous damage to womb
Prolapse of vagina and cervix	Increased abdominal pressure Large litters

Clinical signs	Causes / contributing factors
(Cont.)	Nutritional factors *(Chapter 14)* Old sows Sows housed on sloping floors
Rubbing	Biting flies *(Parasites - Chapter 11)* Dermatitis Harvest mites * Lice or **Mange** * Scurf - dead surface skin
Salivation	Mouth infection Tooth abscesses Vesicular diseases e.g. **FMD** & **SVD** (Section 3) others *(Chapter 12)*
Skin disease/ conditions	Dermatitis **Erysipelas** **Mange** **Porcine reproductive and respiratory syndrome (PRRS)**
Sneezing (Unusual in sows)	Ammonia **Atrophic rhinitis (AR)** * **Aujeszky's disease (AD) (PR)** Bedding (dusty, mouldy) * Cytomegalovirus Virus infections of the nose
Swellings (Joints, muscles, tendons,other)	**Abscesses** **Anthrax** (around the neck) **Erysipelas** **Haematoma** **Glässers disease (Hps)** (Gilts)

Clinical signs	Causes / contributing factors
(Cont.)	**Mycoplasma arthritis** * (Gilts) Ruptured muscle Trauma See also **Lameness**
Thin sows	**Cystitis/pyelonephritis** * Draughts **Eperythrozoonosis (Epe**) Low energy intake * Low environmental temperature * Low feed intake * Old age **Parasites** Poor insulation of buildings Poor nutrition * *(Chapter 14)*
Trembling	**Meningitis** See also nervous symptoms
Ulceration of the skin	**Bush foot / Foot rot** Dermatitis Granuloma (see **Bursitis**) Open wounds Pustular dermatitis *(Chapter 10)* Shoulder sores * Trauma Vesicular diseases (**FMD, SVD** - Sec. 3)
Urine (Chalky mineral deposits or abnormal colour)	**Cystitis / Pyelonephritis** * Nutritional abnormalities *(Chapter 14)* See also blood in urine

Clinical signs	Causes / contributing factors
Vomiting	**Fever** **Gastric ulcers** Gastritis * Over eating Poisons *(Chapter 13)* **Porcine epidemic diarrhoea (PED)** **Transmissible gastro-enteritis (TGE)** **Torsion of the stomach and intestines** **Parasites**
Vulva - abnormal discharges	**Abortion** **Brucellosis** **Cystitis / pyelonephritis** Dead foetuses **Metritis** (Womb infections) * **Peritonitis** Poor environments Vaginitis

* **Most likely**

Lactating Sows

NOTE - If clinical sign is not listed here look in dry sow table

Use the following table to identify the possible cause of disease based on your clinical observations:

Clinical signs	Causes / contributing factors
Abdomen distended (Blown up)	Constipation Dead piglets in womb Excess gas in large bowel * Faulty nutrition Too much food * **Torsion of the stomach and intestines**
Blisters	**Foot and Mouth Disease (FMD)** (Sec. 3) **Swine vesicular disease (SVD)** (Sec. 3) Other vesicular diseases *(Chapter 12)*
Blood from the vulva or vagina	Bleeding from the vagina / womb Dead piglets in womb **Haematoma** * **Navel bleeding** Ruptured blood vessel in womb or vulva * Trauma to vulva
Discolouration of skin Reddening, Blueing (cyanosis)	Acute toxaemia * **Cystitis / pyelonephritis** Dead piglets in womb **Mastitis** - acute * **Metritis** As for Dry Sows
Heavy breathing	Acute infections * e.g. **Mastitis, Metritis** **Anaemia** **Eclampsia**

Clinical signs	Causes / contributing factors
(Cont.)	**Ergot poisoning** (See **Fungal poisoning**) Excess heat Normal at farrowing **Pneumonia** * **Porcine stress syndrome (PSS)** Stress at farrowing *
Mastitis (Agalactia)	Bacterial infections * Damaged teats * **Metritis** Poor floors, hygiene, drainage **Porcine reproductive and respiratory syndrome (PRRS)** Trauma
Mummified piglets	**Aujeszky's disease (AD) (PR)** **Bovine viral diarrhoea (BVD)** Foetal death due to lack of space in the uterus * Leptospirosis Parvovirus * **Porcine reproductive and respiratory syndrome (PRRS)** * **Swine fevers**
No milk / sow will not suckle	Age Discharges Excitation **Fever** **Fungal poisoning** **Mastitis** * **Metritis** (womb infection) *

Clinical signs	Causes / contributing factors
(Cont.)	**Oedema of the udder** * Poor crate design **Porcine reproductive and respiratory syndrome (PRRS)** Shortage of water or **Salt poisoning** Sow ill or toxic * **Swine influenza (SI)** Trauma to teats
Not eating (inappetence) Temperature normal	Specific bacterial infections i.e. nephritis, abscesses Acute toxicaemia * Constipation **Cystitis / pyelonephritis** Dead piglets inside the womb **Gastric ulcers** **Mastitis** **Porcine reproductive and respiratory syndrome (PRRS)** * Water shortage *
Not eating (Inappetence) Temperature elevated	Dead piglets inside the womb **Erysipelas** Farrowing problems Kidney infection **Mastitis** * **Metritis** (womb infection) * **Porcine reproductive and respiratory syndrome (PRRS)** Torsion of the womb Water shortage
Pale pigs	**Anaemia**

Clinical signs	Causes / contributing factors
(Cont.)	**Eperythrozoonosis (Epe)** **Gastric ulcers** * Haemorrhage * As for Dry Sows
Skin diseases / conditions	**Cystitis / pyelonephritis** Dead piglets in womb **Mastitis** - acute *
Udder oedema	Constipation High energy pre farrowing High feed levels pre farrowing * Lack of fibre Shortage of water
Vomiting.	Farrowing on a full stomach As for dry sows

* **Most likely**

PIGLETS

Clinical signs	Causes / contributing factors
Abdomen distended (Blown up)	**Atresia ani -** No rectum * Constipation Excess gas Peritonitis **Torsion of the stomach and intestines** **Vomiting and wasting disease**
Abscesses	Faulty detailing, teeth removal Faulty injections * Trauma to feet, knees, tail *
Anaemia	Copper deficiency **Diarrhoea** - chronic **Eperythrozoonosis (Epe)** Haemorrhage Iron deficiency
Arthritis	See **Lameness**
Blood from the nose	**Atrophic rhinitis (AR) (PAR)** * Trauma *
Blood in faeces	Acute enteritis due to *E. coli* **Clostridial diseases** * **Parasites** **Swine dysentery (SD)** Trauma
Coughing	**Actinobacillosis** **Actinobacillus pleuropneumonia (App)** Dust

Clinical signs	Causes / contributing factors
(Cont.)	Enzootic pneumonia (EP) (usually after 5 weeks) **Glässers disease (Hps)** **Parasites** **Porcine reproductive and respiratory syndrome (PRRS)** * **Swine influenza (SI)** Toxic gases
Dehydration (Sunken eyes, loss of condition)	Bacterial diarrhoea - *E. coli* * **Coccidiosis** **Diarrhoea** **Fever** Haemorrhage **Pneumonia** **Salmonellosis** Shortage of liquids Viral diarrhoea * - **TGE, ED, Rota virus** Vomiting
Diarrhoea 0-5 days of age	**Anaemia** **Clostridial diseases** *E. coli* infections * Low colostrum intake * **Mastitis** * Poor environment **Porcine reproductive and respiratory syndrome (PRRS)** **Rotavirus infection** **Transmissible gastro-enteritis (TGE)** **Udder oedema** and poor milk supply

Clinical signs	Causes / contributing factors
Diarrhoea 6-21 days of age	**Clostridial disease** **Coccidiosis** * **Cryptosporidiosis** * *E. coli* infections Low colostrum intake * Low immunoglobulin A in milk * **Porcine epidemic diarrhoea (PED)** **Porcine reproductive and respiratory syndrome (PRRS)** **Rotavirus infection** **Salmonellosis** Strongyloides *(Chapter 11)* **Transmissible gastro-enteritis (TGE)**
Discharge from eyes.	**Atrophic rhinitis (AR) (PAR)** * Cytomegalo virus **Porcine reproductive and respiratory syndrome (PRRS)** *
Discharge from nose	**Atrophic rhinitis (AR) (PAR)** * **Bordetellosis** (Section 3) Rhinitis
Discolouration of skin (Reddening, Blueing)	**Actinobacillosis** **Actinobacillus pleuropneumonia (App)** **Erysipelas** **Fever** **Glässers disease (Hps)** **Porcine reproductive and respiratory syndrome (PRRS)**
Dog sitting position	Acute arthritis Fractured spine

Clinical signs	Causes / contributing factors
(Cont.)	**Splay legs** * Trauma
Fever - increased temperature	Actinobacillus suis infections **Erysipelas** (rarely) **Glässers disease (Hps)** Specific bacteria diseases * **Streptococcal infections** (Section 3)
Fits - convulsions Frothing at mouth	**Aujeszky's disease (AD) (PR)** **Glässers disease (Hps)** **Hypoglycaemia** * **Meningitis** **Salt poisoning (Water deprivation)** **Swine fevers** See also nervous symptoms
Greasy skin	**Greasy pig disease** * Poor nutrition **Porcine reproductive and respiratory syndrome (PRRS)** Pustular dermatitis *(Chapter 10)* Shortage of essential fatty acids
Haemorrhage	See blood Enteritis * **Navel bleeding** * Trauma
Hairiness	**Arthritis** * Chilling **Diarrhoea** * **Fever**

Clinical signs	Causes / contributing factors
(Cont.)	**Hypoglycaemia** **Meningitis**
Head on one side or shaking	**Aujeszky's disease (AD) (PR)** Encephalitis **Glässers disease (Hps)** **Meningitis** **Middle ear infection** *
Heavy breathing	**Anaemia** Heat stroke Septicaemia / **fever** See also **Pneumonia**
Jaundice - yellow skin	**Leptospirosis** * **Anaemia** **Eperythrozoonosis (Epe)**
Jerky eye movements -Nystagmus	**Aujeszky's disease (AD) (PR)** **Glässers disease (Hps)** **Meningitis** *
Laid on / trauma	Inadequate temperatures Poor crate design Poor environment Poor farrowing house design Poor farrowing house management **Splay legs**
Lameness	*Actinobacillus suis* infections **Arthritis** **Erysipelas** Faulty teeth clipping and or tailing *

Clinical signs	Causes / contributing factors
(Cont.)	**Fractures** **Glässers disease (Hps)** Navel infection Poor environment particularly floor surfaces * Shivering Specific infections **Splaylegs** Staphylococci Streptococci * Trauma to knees, tail etc. * Vitamin E / Iron toxicity
Meningitis	**Aujeszky's disease (AD) (PR)** **Glässers disease (Hps)** * **Streptococcal infections** * (Section 3) **Swine fevers** See also nervous signs
Mortality - Generalised infection	*Actinobacillus suis* infections **Aujeszky's disease (AD) (PR)** *E. coli* infections * **Eperythrozoonosis (Epe)** **Erysipelas** **Glässers disease (Hps)** **Meningitis** **Porcine reproductive and respiratory syndrome (PRRS)** **Swine influenza (SI)**
Mortality - Good pigs found dead	Acute enteritis Defective heart Laid on *

Clinical signs	Causes / contributing factors
(Cont.)	No colostrum * Pale pigs **Diarrhoea or scour** Septicaemia Starvation Stillborn Trauma
Mortality - Trauma	Laid on
Mortality - due to poor viability	**Agalactia** - No milk in the sow * Age or breed of the sow **Diarrhoea** **Swine influenza** infection during pregnancy **Hypoglycaemia** (low blood sugar) Hypothermia - chilling **Leptospirosis** Low birth weight * **Mastitis** in the sow and lack of milk * **Navel bleeding** Poor colostrum intake Poor environment Poor management * Poor nutrition / starvation **Porcine reproductive and respiratory syndrome (PRRS)** **Porcine reproductive and respiratory syndrome (PRRS)** in the sow **Splay legs** **Thrombocytopaenic purpura** (bleeding) **Udder oedema** in the sow and no milk

Clinical signs	Causes / contributing factors
Mortality - sudden	**Actinobacillosis** Acute enteritis (*E. coli*) **Clostridial diseases** * **Glässers disease (Hps**) Iron toxicity **Meningitis** **Navel bleeding** **Thrombocytopaenic purpura** **Torsion of the stomach and intestines** Trauma
Mummified piglets *(Chapter 6)*	**Aujeszky's disease (AD) (PR)** Foetal death due to lack of space in the uterus * **Leptospirosis** **Porcine parvovirus (PPV)** * **Porcine reproductive and respiratory syndrome (PRRS)** * **Swine fevers**
Muscle trembling	**Congenital tremor (CT)** * **Hypoglycaemia** **Meningitis** **Swine fevers, Tetanus**
Nervous symptoms e.g. Fits Blindness Muscle tremors Paralysis Loss of balance Lameness Paddling on side	**Actinobacillosis** **Aujeszky's disease (AD) (PR)** **Congenital tremor (CT)** * **Glässers disease (Hps)** Hypoglycaemia * Iron toxicity **Middle ear infection** **Porcine reproductive and respiratory**

Clinical signs	Causes / contributing factors
(Cont.)	**syndrome (PRRS)** Streptococcal meningitis **Swine fevers** **Tetanus** Trauma
Not suckling	**Diarrhoea** **Fever** **Lameness**
Pain	**Arthritis** **Meningitis**
Pale pigs	Acute enteritis **Anaemia** * **Clostridial disease** **Eperythrozoonosis (Epe)** Faulty detailing, teeth removal Faulty injections. **Glässers disease (Hps)** Haemorrhage **Leptospirosis** **Vitamin E deficiency and Iron Toxicity** **Navel bleeding** * Shortage of iron * **Thrombocytopaenic purpura** Trauma, Trauma to feet
Paralysis	**Aujeszky's disease (AD) (PR)** **Brucellosis** **Hypoglycaemia** Streptococcal infections Trauma

Clinical signs	Causes / contributing factors
Pneumonia	**Actinobacillosis** **Glässers disease (Hps)** Septicaemia * **Streptococcal infections** (Section 3)
Poor viability	**Aujeszky's disease (AD) (PR)** **Agalactia** - no milk in the sow Chilling **Hypoglycaemia** (low blood sugar) * Hypothermia * **Leptospirosis** Low birth weight * No milk * **Porcine Parvovirus (PPV)** **Porcine reproductive and respiratory syndrome (PRRS)** infection in the sow See also **Mortality**
Shivering	**Fever** Joint infections * **Meningitis** * **Hypoglycaemia** * Vomiting **Diarrhoea or scour** *
Skin diseases / conditions	**Erysipelas** **Greasy pig disease** **Mange** **Porcine reproductive and respiratory syndrome (PRRS)**
Sneezing	**Actinobacillus pleuropneumonia (App)** Ammonia

Clinical signs	Causes / contributing factors
(Cont.)	**Atrophic rhinitis (AR)** * **Aujeszky's disease (AD) (PR)** Bedding (dusty, mouldy) **Bordetellosis** (Section 3) Dust **Enzootic pneumonia (EP)** **Glässers disease (Hps)** Poor environments * Porcine cytomegalovirus (PCMV) **Porcine reproductive and respiratory syndrome (PRRS)** **Swine influenza (SI)** Virus infections of the nose
Starvation / wasting	See poor viable piglets *Actinobacillus suis* infections **Anaemia** **Arthritis** Chronic **diarrhoea** * **Coccidiosis** **Congenital tremor (CT)** **Eperythrozoonosis (Epe)** Low birth weight No milk available * **Pneumonia** Poor colostrum intake * Poor environment Poor teat access * **Porcine reproductive and respiratory syndrome (PRRS)** *
Stillborn piglets	Age of sow **Aujeszky's disease (AD) (PR)**

Clinical signs	Causes / contributing factors
(Cont.)	Born alive but found dead Enterovirus **Erysipelas** **Fever** in sows Haemorrhage, septicaemia, stress, anaemia High house temperatures Large litters * **Leptospirosis** **Porcine Parvovirus (PPV)** **Porcine reproductive and respiratory syndrome (PRRS)**
Swellings (joints, muscles or tendons, others)	*Actinobacillus suis* infections **Bursitis** Faulty teeth / tail clipping **Glässers disease (Hps)** Navel infections Scrubbed knees **Streptococcal infections** * (Section 3) Trauma Faulty iron injections **Fractures** **Haematoma** Infected gums Rupture
Trembling	**Congenital tremor (CT)** * **Meningitis** See also nervous symptoms
Vomiting	Constipation *E. coli* infections *

Clinical signs	Causes / contributing factors
(Cont.)	Gastritis * **Heat stroke** Injections of penicillin **Swine fevers** **Transmissible gastro-enteritis (TGE)** * **Vomiting wasting disease**

* **Most likely**

Abortion

(Abortion is covered in detail in Chapters 5 and 6).

Embryo loss and abortion

Embryo loss occurs when there is death of embryos followed by absorption, or expulsion.

Abortion means the premature expulsion of dead or non-viable foetuses.

Records help to identify reproductive problems.

These should include information on:

- Age (or parity) profile of the herd.
- Failure to come on heat.
- Culling rates.
- Bleeding and discharges from the vulva.
- Repeats, sows not in pig.
- Lameness.
- Litter sizes.
- Mastitis, lack of milk, swollen udders.
- Deaths and their likely causes.
- Poor conformation.
- Prolapse of the vagina or rectum.
- Savaging.

Symptoms

☞ Mucus, blood, pus discharges from the vulva.

☞ Sow may be ill or normal.

☞ Symptoms of a specific disease.

Causes

Infectious Causes (common ones). Consider the following:

- Aujeszky's disease.
- Influenza virus.
- PRRS (Blue ear disease).
- Leptospira.
- Specific bacteria, *E. coli,* klebsiella, streptococci, pseudomonas.
- Parasite burdens.
- Cystitis, nephritis.

Non Infectious Causes

- Seasonal infertility.
- Decreasing daylight length, poor lighting.
- Low temperatures.
- Chilling, draughts.
- Poor nutrition.
- Mouldy feeds.
- Contaminated water.
- Stress.
- No boar contact.
- Vaccine reaction.
- Lameness.
- Poor hygiene.

Diagnosis

Fresh, aborted foetuses should be submitted to a competent diagnostic laboratory where examinations can be carried out for evidence of viral and bacterial infections, together with histological examinations and toxic studies. In many cases the end results of post-mortem and serological tests do not identify any particular infectious organism, which may seem disappointing. However, it is useful in telling us what is not present.

A Checklist for Abortions

1. Abortion Level. Is this more than 1.5% of sows served? - Take action.
2. Are sows ill?
   - Probably disease.
3. Are sows otherwise normal?
   - Probably non infectious
   - Maternal failures.
4. Is the problem seasonal?
   - Autumn abortion syndrome.
5. Do they occur in a particular part of the farm?
   - Environmental.
6. Are the aborted pigs fresh or alive?

- Suggests the environment.

7. Are mummified pigs present?
   - Suggests infection.
8. Is the dry sow accommodation uncomfortable?
   -Suggests the environment.
9. Are sow pens wet, draughty, poorly lit?
   - Suggests the environment.
10. Does the ventilation system chill the sows?
   - Suggests the environment.
11. Are there factors that place the sows in a negative energy state? e.g.:High chill factors, draughts, low feed intake, a change in bedding, availability.
12. Are sows short of food - Check feed intakes by volume and weight.
13. Is the food mouldy?
   - Check for mouldy feed.
14. Do the sows experience 14 hours of good light at eye level?
15. Are the lights dirty, covered in fly dirt?
16. Can you read a newspaper in the darkest corner?
17. Do your sows have boar contact in pregnancy?
18. Are any other diseases evident in the sows?
   e.g.: lameness , cystitis, kidney infections.
19. Are the abortions associated with stress?
20. Increase feed intake from days 3 to 21 after mating according to body condition and environmental temperatures.
21. Increase the mating programme by 10-15% over the anticipated period of infertility.
22. Because boar semen can be affected, follow each natural mating 24 hours later by purchased AI.

Abscesses

(Chapter 10 pp352)

Pockets of pus that contain large numbers of bacteria which usually enter the body through damage to the skin. Near the skin surface they may become painful.

Symptoms

<u>All Pigs</u>

- ☞ Possibly emaciation and death.
- ☞ Small to large swellings.

Causes / Contributing factors

- Fighting.
- Secondary infection to other conditions such as PRRS, pneumonia or tail biting.
- Small widespread abscesses in the skin (pustular dermatitis) may be seen following general illness, septicaemia and or greasy pig disease.
- Damage to the skin by sharp objects in the environment.
- Trauma to feet, knees, tail.
- Teeth removal.

Diagnosis

Feel and press the swelling to ascertain if the contents are fluid or solid. Sample the contents by inserting an 18mm 16 gauge needle attached to a 10ml syringe at the lowest soft point of the swelling.

Haemorrhage into the tissues is the only condition likely to be confused with an abscess. In such cases either pure blood or a very thin blood stained liquid will be withdrawn. Such pockets of blood are called haematomas.

Treatment

- ❒ Test the contents with a needle and syringe - blood or pus.
- ❒ Drain the pus by making an incision with a sharp scalpel blade approximately 15-20mm long at the lowest point particularly where it feels soft. Sometimes drainage will occur spontaneously after the abscess bursts.
- ❒ Squeeze into the hole an antibiotic cream (a cow mastitis tube is ideal) containing penicillin/streptomycin, oxytetracycline, amoxycillin or ampicillin or give an intramuscular injection of penicillin.

Actinobacillosis

(Chapter 8 pp258)

This is caused by the bacteria, *Actinobacillus suis* and *Actinobacillus equuli.* The first of these is present in most herds and lives in the tonsils of older pigs, particularly sows. It usually only effects piglets.

Symptoms

Sows

- ☞ Rarely applicable.

Piglets

- ☞ Sudden death.
- ☞ Discoloration of skin.
- ☞ High fever.
- ☞ Coughing.
- ☞ Pneumonia.
- ☞ Skin lesions (not to be confused with Erysipelas).
- ☞ Arthritis.
- ☞ Lameness.
- ☞ Septicaemia.

Causes / Contributing factors

- It can be precipitated by PRRS.
- Teeth clipping .
- De-tailing.
- Scrubbed knees.
- It may enter the piglet via the respiratory system or via cuts and abrasions.
- It occasionally multiplies in the blood stream and settles out in various parts of the body, particularly the lungs and the joints. Here it produces multiple small abscesses.

Diagnosis

Post-mortem laboratory examination to demonstrate characteristic lesions and the presence of the organism. It has to be differentiated from meningitis, acute *E. coli* infection, erysipelas, clostridial diseases and piglets that have been laid on.

Treatment

❒ The organism is sensitive to most antibiotics but in particular amoxycillin or ampicillin injected at 5mg per kg or procaine penicillin, 1ml/20kg.

❒ In persistent outbreaks if the onset of the disease is predictable preventive measures can be taken by giving long-acting preparations of antibiotics to all litters over a period of 3 to 4 weeks.

❒ In-feed medication of the sow with phenoxymethyl penicillin at 200g/tonne for the first 3 weeks after farrowing has proved successful in problem cases.

Actinobacillus Pleuropneumonia (App)

This is similar in all pigs - see Section 3.

Agalactia - No Milk

(Chapter 8 pp239)

This is a failure of milk let down, shortage of milk or no milk in an otherwise healthy animal.

Symptoms

Lactating Sows only

☞ Inappetence.

☞ May have slight fever.

☞ Udder tissue is poorly developed and disappearing.

Causes / Contributing factors

- Old age.
- Excess body condition.
- Water shortage.
- Poor crate design.
- Sequel to oedema or mastitis.

Diagnosis

This is based upon the appearance of the litter, piglets showing starvation, and the udder which lacks milk and is "drying up".

Treatment

❒ There will be no response to treatment. Cull the sow

ANAEMIA

(Chapter 8 pp259)

This is mainly a disease of the piglet because it is born with limited supplies of iron a vital component in blood cells. If the piglet does not have access to iron in the first 2 - 3 weeks it's red cell capacity to absorb oxygen (anaemia) is impaired.

Symptoms

Sows (Growing Pigs)

- ☞ Pale (but well grown).
- ☞ Breathless on exertion.

Piglets

- ☞ Pale.
- ☞ Breathless on exertion.
- ☞ Jaundiced sometimes(Skin slight yellow appearance).
- ☞ Mucous membranes of the eyes are pale.
- ☞ Scour.

Causes / Contributing factors

It can arise in one of three ways:

1. Loss of blood through haemorrhage.
2. Dietary insufficiencies, particularly iron and copper.
3. Disease - infection or poisoning (e.g. warfarin, parasites).

Diagnosis

This is based on the clinical signs, the lack of any supplemental iron and the haemoglobin level of less than 8g/100ml in the blood.

Treatment

- ❒ Give an injection of iron dextran. 1000mg per sow.
- ❒ The piglet is born with limited supplies of iron. The easiest method of prevention is to give the piglet an injection of 150-200mg of iron dextran in either a 1 or 2ml dose.
- ❒ Iron is best given from 3 to 5 days of age and not at birth, when it may cause unnecessary trauma to the muscles.
- ❒ Carry out regular worming programmes.
- ❒ Specific treatment will depend on the cause.

ANTHRAX

(Chapter 7 pp200)

This is an uncommon disease of pigs in most parts of the world. Care should be taken in handling diseased pigs or carcasses because anthrax is communicable to people. Effective vaccines are available in some countries for both pigs and people.

Symptoms

<u>All Pigs</u>

- ☞ Acute illness.
- ☞ Fever.
- ☞ Respiratory distress.
- ☞ Sudden death.
- ☞ Swollen throat.

Causes / Contributing factors

- ◆ The source of the infection in sows is usually contaminated feed.

Diagnosis

Anthrax should be suspected if a sow is found dead and post-mortem examination shows copious blood tinged tissue fluid and large red lymph nodes under the skin of the neck and in the abdomen. The post-mortem examination should be discontinued immediately and veterinary help sought.

Treatment

- ❒ Penicillin by injection.
- ❒ Vaccination is possible.

ARTHRITIS - JOINT INFECTIONS

(Chapter 8 pp260 and Chapter 9 pp317)

This is common in all sucking and growing pigs, the causes are mainly bacteria. The bacteria include *Actinobacillus suis, Haemophilus parasuis, E. coli*, staphylococci, and streptococci. The commonest in sucking pigs is *Streptococcus suis* type 1 which causes chronic lesions sporadically in individual pigs but *Streptococcus suis* type 14, which is less common, also causes severe sudden outbreaks of very painful arthritis. Mycoplasma arthritis is rare in piglets. Erysipelas is uncommon due to the presence of maternal antibody but as this disappears from between 6 - 10 weeks of age disease may develop.

Symptoms

<u>Sows</u>

- ☞ Lameness.
- ☞ Stiffness.

<u>Piglets</u>

- ☞ Shivering.
- ☞ Lameness pain.
- ☞ Reluctance to rise.
- ☞ Hairy appearance.
- ☞ Swollen hock and elbow joints.
- ☞ Stiffness or lameness.

Causes / Contributing factors

Mainly piglets

- ◆ Trauma.
- ◆ Knee necrosis.
- ◆ Faulty iron injections.
- ◆ Poor floor surfaces.
- ◆ Faulty teeth clipping, tail docking, worn equipment.
- ◆ Navel infection.

Diagnosis

Based on lameness and the swollen joints but laboratory culture is required to identify the organism.

Treatment

- ❒ Using one of the following antibiotics: lincomycin, penicillin and streptomycin, oxytetracycline, amoxycillin, ampicillin, trimethoprim/sulpha, enrofloxacin or framycetin, is only effective if given very early. Inject daily for five days. Long-acting preparations can also be used and these should be injected every other day. Antibiotic penetration of the joint is slow.

Atresia ani - No Anus or No Rectum

(Chapter 8 pp261)

The piglet is born with a blind end to its rectum, 5-10mm in length with no anus. It is not worth attempting surgical repair. Death invariably ensues. The incidence in mature herds is usually less than 0.5% but it can be much higher in newly established gilt herds. The condition is heritable but of low penetrance. Records may indicate that a certain boar is involved. The abdomens of affected piglets becomes enlarged. Some piglets may survive to weaning. Affected piglets should be destroyed.

Atrophic Rhinitis (AR) Progressive Atrophic Rhinitis (PAR)

(Chapter 8 pp261)

Rhinitis is inflammation of the tissues inside the nose and in its mild form its very common. This condition rarely causes clinical disease in the mature animal but if the breeding female has been infected early in life it could still show distortions of the face in adulthood. Progressive atrophic rhinitis is a serious condition both in sucking and growing pigs. The term atrophy indicates that the tissues inside the nose, which become infected or damaged, shrink and become distorted. There are two forms of the disease: mild and non-progressive where the infection or irritation occurs over a period of 2 to 3 weeks. However, the inflammation does not progress and structures in the nose called turbinate bones repair and return to normality.

The serious disease is progressive atrophic rhinitis (PAR) where toxin producing strains of the bacterium *Pasteurella multocidia*, present in the herd cause a continual and progressive inflammation and atrophy of the tissues and nose distortion. All herds will show some degree of non-progressive atrophic rhinitis.

Symptoms

Sows

- None clinically.
- Distortion of the face.

Piglets

- Sneezing.
- Runny eyes.
- Discharges from the nose, sometimes containing blood.
- Distortion of the face.
- Shortening or twisting of the upper jaw.

Causes / Contributing factors

- More common in young herds particularly those containing

large numbers of gilts.

- Large permanently populated farrowing houses.
- Multi suckling increases the spread of infection.
- Poor ventilation, low humidity.
- Dusty atmospheres predispose.
- Toxic gases predispose.
- The presence of diseases such as PRRS, Hps and Aujeszky's disease.

Diagnosis

Clinical signs in sucking piglets. Sneezing is common in sucking piglets and need not necessarily be associated with PAR. Individual piglets may also develop distortion of the nose from trauma or some cause other than PAR. Swabbing the nostril and submitting to a specialist laboratory for examination. Post-mortem examination of the nose.

Treatment

- ❐ Vaccinate the complete breeding herd immediately.
- ❐ In-feed medicate sows with trimethoprim/sulpha or sulphadimidine from point of entry into farrowing through to weaning.
- ❐ Inject all piglets with 0.25 to 0.5ml of long acting OTC or amoxycillin on days 3, 10 and 15 during sucking.
- ❐ Inject pigs similarly at weaning time with 0.5 to 1ml of long acting antibiotic.
- ❐ Medicate the creep rations with OTC or CTC 800g/tonne or trimethoprim/sulpha combinations for 4 weeks post weaning.
- ❐ Vaccination of breeding females is effective in reducing the carrier state and preventing infection of the sow's offspring.

Aujeszky's disease (AD) / Pseudorabies (PR)

(Chapter 6 pp167 and Chapter 12 pp396)

This is an important disease of pigs caused by a herpes virus. Once introduced into a herd the virus usually remains there and it can continually affect reproductive performance at varying levels. The virus can survive for up to three weeks outside the pig. Acute outbreaks of disease occur when virulent strains of the virus first infect an unvaccinated susceptible herd. The virus crosses the uterus and placenta and infects the foetuses.

Symptoms

Dry Sow

- ☞ Coughing.
- ☞ Nervous signs.
- ☞ Reproductive failure.
- ☞ Abortions.
- ☞ Mummified piglets.
- ☞ Stillbirths.
- ☞ Birth weak litters.

Piglets

- ☞ Nervous signs.
- ☞ Incoordination.
- ☞ Sneezing.
- ☞ Coughing.
- ☞ High mortality.

All Other Species

- ☞ Nervous signs.
- ☞ Death.

Causes / Contributing factors

- Movement of carrier pigs.
- Virus airborne - at least 3km (2 miles).
- Infection from feral (wild) pigs.
- The role of mechanical spread by birds is questionable.
- Contaminated carcasses may spread infection.
- Mechanically on people.
- Contaminated vehicles.
- Through infected semen via AI or a carrier boar.
- From infected slurry.

Diagnosis

When a susceptible breeding herd first breaks down with this disease the clinical signs described above strongly suggest aujeszky's disease and are almost diagnostic. Laboratory tests are required to confirm the diagnosis.

Treatment

- ❒ None is available but antibiotic medication to control secondary bacteria in a new outbreak could be considered.
- ❒ 600-800g of CTC or OTC in the breeding ration for 3-4 weeks as advised by the veterinarian.
- ❒ **Vaccination**. This is the key action to take. As soon as disease

is identified all breeding stock should be vaccinated with a gene deleted vaccine to mitigate the effects and reduce spread of the virus. Disease can be eliminated.

- ❐ Gilts and boars should only be purchased from known free herds and be vaccinated before arrival or in isolation.
- ❐ Keep disease out of the herd by isolating all purchased breeding stock and blood sampling them before they enter the herd.
- ❐ If your herd is at risk, in other words within a 3km radius of large infected herds, then vaccinate it to prevent disease.

BACK MUSCLE NECROSIS

(Chapter 7 pp201)

Back muscle necrosis is part of the porcine stress syndrome and in affected pigs degenerative changes take place in the back muscles along each side of the spine. It is usually seen in the young growing gilt although occasionally it occurs in the adult female. The disease is relatively uncommon.

Symptoms

Young Growing Pigs and Gilts

- ☞ The symptoms are sudden in onset after exercise.
- ☞ Severe pain in the lumber muscles with obvious swellings.
- ☞ Death (necrosis) of muscle fibres with haemorrhages into the tissues themselves.
- ☞ Reluctant to stand.
- ☞ Adopt a dog sitting position.
- ☞ The temperature is usually normal but may be elevated.
- ☞ Discoloration of the skin over the affected area.

Causes / Contributing factors

- ◆ Sudden movement e.g. from confinement to outdoor accommodation.
- ◆ Presence of the halothane gene.

Diagnosis

Based on the clinical signs. The pig can be made to stand with difficulty but there is no evidence of fractures. Examine the lumber muscles carefully, they will be swollen and painful on pressure. History includes sudden lameness associated with movement and acute pain.

Treatment

❒ Inject with phenylbutazone 1ml/50kg or other pain killer.
❒ Inject with corticosteroids provided the animal is not pregnant.
❒ If there is a temperature give an injection of long-acting penicillin to cover the possibility of erysipelas.

Biotin Deficiency

(Chapter 7 pp201)

Biotin is present in most nutrient sources and deficiency is unlikely. The role of biotin in nutrition and the changes that result when it is deficient are not clear. Reports and field studies however have highlighted the following associations.

Symptoms

Sows	Piglets
☞ Lameness throughout the herd or a group of sows.	☞ N/A
☞ Laminitis.	
☞ Hooves will be soft over the walls.	
☞ Haemorrhage over the solar surfaces of the feet.	
☞ Dark transverse cracks in hooves.	
☞ Excessive hair loss.	
☞ Extended weaning to mating intervals.	
☞ Poor litter size.	

Causes / Contributing factors

- Biotin deficiency in the diet.
- Possible cause trauma from poor floor surfaces.

Diagnosis

Based on the clinical picture and the fact that the herd or a group of animals will be affected. Chronic lesions of swine vesicular disease could be confused with biotin deficiency.

Treatment

❒ Where a herd shows widespread lesions add up to 0.5-1mg/kg to the diet. Response will take up to 9 months.
❒ Add biotin to the diet as a routine.

❐ Occasionally lameness problems caused by soft hooves with dark transverse cracks appear to be improved with biotin supplementation of the diet; 100-200mg/tonne is adequate.

Bordetellosis

This is similar in all pigs see Section 3.

Botulism

Bacteria called clostridia produce toxins (poisons). *Clostridium botulinium,* which produces this disease grows in decaying vegetable matter producing the toxin which is then eaten. However botulism is rare in pigs. It should be considered as a food poisoning.

Symptoms

These are seen 4-48 hours or so after the toxin has been eaten.

<u>All Pigs</u>

☞ Muscle paralysis.
☞ Weakness of limbs leading to complete paralysis.
☞ Blindness.
☞ Excessive salivation.
☞ Loss of bladder function.
☞ Breathing difficulties.

Causes / Contributing factors

- Decaying feed.
- Contaminated water or feed.

Diagnosis

This is based on the symptoms, evidence of decomposing food and demonstration of the presence of toxin by a laboratory .

Treatment

❐ There is no specific treatment.

Bovine Viral Diarrhoea Virus (BVD) and Border Disease (BD)

(Chapter 6 pp168)

There are two viruses, which are in the same group of pestiviruses as the virus of swine fever (hog cholera) but which primarily infect cattle and sheep respectively. They can get into pig breeding herds and cause reproductive problems.

The disease is not a common cause of infertility in the sow and would be considered low on the list of possibilities from a diagnostic point of view.

Symptoms

<u>Sows</u>
- ☞ Poor conception rates.
- ☞ A few abortions.
- ☞ Foetal death.
- ☞ Mummification.
- ☞ Small litters.
- ☞ Low birth weights.

<u>Piglets</u>
- ☞ N/A

Causes / Contributing factors

- Exposure of pigs to cattle or sheep faeces.
- Feeding of un-pasteurised cow's milk, or in contaminated live-attenuated virus vaccines.

Diagnosis

Laboratory tests.

Treatment

- ❒ There is no treatment and the infections are self eliminating.

BRUCELLOSIS

(Chapter 12 pp401)

This disease is caused by the bacterium *Brucella suis*, which is one of the six different species of brucella. *Brucella suis* does not exist in the UK, Ireland and in some other EU countries, Canada and most states of the USA but is widespread through most of the rest of the pig rearing world. It is an important disease not least because some strains of it can be transmitted to people and is serious. A carrier state persists for long periods of time.

Symptoms

<u>Sows</u>
- ☞ Bacteraemia (bacteria in the blood).
- ☞ Infertility.

<u>Piglets</u>
- ☞ Paralysis of hind legs.

☞ Abortions at any time.
☞ Vulval discharges.
☞ Delayed returns.
☞ Swollen/ painful testicles (boar).

Causes / Contributing factors

- Spread by venereal infection.
- The boar is a major source either by direct contact at mating or via artificial insemination.
- Pigs can also be infected via the conjunctiva, through the nose or by mouth.
- The hare in Northern Europe can also be infected and is considered a natural host.
- Carrier sows.

Diagnosis

This can be readily carried out by isolation of the organism. Serology is used to detect carrier sows but cross reactions can occur quite extensively due to another organism called *Yersinia enterocolitica*. If the serum agglutination test (SAT) is used results of 31 international units (iu) or more are considered positive. The complement fixation test (CFT) is often used in conjunction with the SAT for export testing purposes.

Treatment

❒ Is not effective. Antibiotics give a poor response.
❒ Depopulate the herd.

Bursitis

(Chapter 7 pp202)

Bursitis is a common condition in all pigs. A soft lump arises from repeated pressure and trauma to the skin overlying any bony prominence. It can commence in piglets in the farrowing houses, particularly if there are bad floors, but it usually starts in the weaner accommodation on slatted floors which have large gaps. Wire mesh, woven metal and metal bar floors can produce high levels in weaner pigs in first and second stage housing. If the lumps remain uninfected the condition commercially is not important but if breeding stock is being produced, rejection rates may be high.

Symptoms

All Pigs

- ☞ Swellings develop on the hocks and elbows.
- ☞ Infection may occur.
- ☞ If skin is broken and secondary infection occurs abscesses develop.
- ☞ Ulceration of the skin.
- ☞ Lameness.

Causes / Contributing factors

- ◆ Poor floor surfaces.
- ◆ Lack of bedding.
- ◆ High stocking densities.
- ◆ Bad slats in confinement.

Treatment

- ❒ There is no specific treatment.
- ❒ Most lesions do not require treatment.
- ❒ If the swellings have become infected with bacteria inject with either oxytetracycline or ampicillin.
- ❒ If *Mycoplasma hyosynoviae* is causing infection use either lincomycin or tiamulin.
- ❒ Remove pigs to well bedded pens.
- ❒ Determine the point at which lesions are occurring.

Bush Foot / Foot Rot

(Chapter 7 pp202)

Bush foot results from infection of the claw which becomes swollen and painful around the coronary band. It arises through penetration of the sole of the foot, cracks at the sole-hoof junction, or splitting of the hoof itself. It usually occurs in one foot only and is more commonly seen in the hind feet especially the outer claws, which are the larger ones carrying proportionately more weight. Infection sometimes penetrates the soft tissues between the claws and this is referred to as foot rot. The claw becomes enlarged and inflamed. Lameness in sows and boars may lower reproductive performance.

See *Chapter 7 pp209* for other causes of lameness.

Symptoms

<u>All Pigs</u>

- ☞ Lameness.
- ☞ Painful swollen claw.
- ☞ Cracks at the sole-hoof junction, or splitting of the hoof itself.
- ☞ As the infection progresses inside the hoof, the claw becomes enlarged and infection and inflammation of the joint often develops.
- ☞ In most cases a swelling is visible around the coronary band which may form an abscess and burst to the surface.

Causes / Contributing factors

- ◆ It arises through penetration of the sole of the foot.
- ◆ Cracks at the sole-hoof junction, or splitting of the hoof itself.
- ◆ Poor floor surfaces.
- ◆ Trauma to piglets from the sow.
- ◆ Trauma to piglets from slatted floors.

Diagnosis

This is based on the clinical signs. Bush foot has to be differentiated from other forms of trauma and infection including erysipelas, glässers disease, leg weakness or osteochondrosis (OCD) and mycoplasma arthritis.

Treatment

- ❒ Antibiotics which can be used, depending on the advice of your veterinarian, include:

- Lincocin	11mg/kg liveweight.
- Oxytetracycline	25 mg/kg liveweight.
- Amoxycillin	15mg/kg liveweight.

- ❒ Inject daily for 5 to 7 days.
  If there is no improvement in three days change the antibiotic.
  Complete recovery may take 3-4 weeks.
- ❒ Anti-inflammatory injections of cortisone may be given provided the sow is not pregnant.
- ❒ An anti-inflammatory drug such as phenylbutazone may be administered either by mouth or injection.

- ❐ If there is a herd problem a foot bath containing either 1% formalin (only use in the open air) or 5% copper sulphate will help. Walk the sows through once each week on 2-3 occasions. However if there are dry cracked claws in the herd, this treatment might make them worse.

Clostridial Diseases

(Chapter 7 pp203 and Chapter 8 pp263)

Clostridia are large gram-positive spore-bearing bacteria that are present in the large intestine of all pigs. There are several species. They multiply rapidly and produce toxins that rapidly kill the host. This disease can be a major problem in outdoor breeding pigs (*C. novyi*). The organisms may enter the body through damage to the skin and underlying tissues and muscles. Bacterial spores also get carried from their normal habitat, the gut, to the liver where they may lie latent and inactive for long periods. The course of the disease is extremely short and often the only sign is a dead pig.

The disease caused by *C. perfringens* type A tends to be milder, less dramatic and more prolonged but it can look similar to that caused by type C.

Clostridial disease in the sow during lactation is not common.

The most common disease in sows is associated with *C. novyi* which causes sudden death. Whenever sow mortality rises above 4%, this disease should be considered.

The species, *C. perfringens*, types A, B or C, can under certain conditions produce a severe diarrhoea with very high mortality in piglets. Type C is by far the most important and if it gets into the small intestine and becomes established before colostrum is taken in, disease can result. Piglets are normally infected under 7 days of age and more typically within the first 24 to 72 hours of life.

Symptoms

Sows

- ☞ Sudden death.
- ☞ Gangrene, characterised by

Piglets

- ☞ Rotten smelling diarrhoea often blood coloured.

painful and discoloured swellings.
- ☞ Fluid and gas are often present in the tissues.

- ☞ Diarrhoea 0-5 days of age.
- ☞ Diarrhoea 6-21 days of age
- ☞ The lining of the small intestine sloughs off (necrosis) and may be observed in the scour.
- ☞ Many piglets die.
- ☞ Bubble of gas in the small intestines.

Causes / Contributing factors

- ◆ High numbers of bacteria in the environment.
- ◆ Unknown factors.
- ◆ Trauma to muscles.
- ◆ Immuno suppressive diseases e.g. PRRS, fungal poisoning.

Diagnosis

In acute cases diagnosis is by the clinical signs and post-mortem lesions, which are diagnostic. It is necessary to submit preferably a live or very recently dead pig to the laboratory (within 3 to 4 hours) because the causal organisms multiply after death and cause rapid post-mortem changes. If the abdomen of a dead pig is cut open the middle portion of the small intestine is often claret wine coloured. A characteristic feature is the very rapid post-mortem change particularly in the liver, which is full of gas and turns a chocolate colour. Confirmation of the diagnosis must be carried out in a laboratory by a fluorescent antibody test to identify the bacterium.

Treatment

<u>Sow</u>

- ❒ Clostridia are very sensitive to penicillin.
- ❒ In-feed medication using 200 grams to the tonne of phenoxymethyl penicillin can be used for 3-4 weeks to control acute outbreaks whilst a vaccination programme is established.
- ❒ Long-acting injections of penicillin given in anticipation of disease may help in the short term.

<u>Piglets</u>

- ❒ In acute outbreaks antiserum can sometimes be helpful when injected into the piglets at birth.

- ❒ Oral antibiotics and in particular amoxycillin should be given at birth and again at day 2 or 3.
- ❒ The sows ration can be medicated with 200g/tonne of phenoxymethyl penicillin or the feed top dressed daily with the premix, from 5 days pre-farrowing and during lactation.

Coccidiosis (Coccidia)

(Chapter 8 pp263)

Coccidiosis is caused by small parasites that multiply inside the host cells, mainly in the intestinal tract. There are three types, Eimeria, Isospora and Cryptosporidia.

Disease is common and widespread in sucking piglets and occasionally in pigs up to 15 weeks of age.

Coccidiosis should be suspected if there is a diarrhoea problem in sucking pigs from 7-21 days of age that does not respond particularly well to antibiotics.

Symptoms

Sows

- ☞ None.
- ☞ Sows are carriers.

Piglets

- ☞ Diarrhoea is the main clinical sign.
- ☞ The faeces vary in consistency and colour from yellow to grey green, or bloody according to the severity of the condition.
- ☞ Dehydration is common.
- ☞ Starvation / Wasting.

Causes / Contributing factors

- Dirty pens.
- Poor hygiene in farrowing pens.
- Poor wet floor surfaces.
- Creep feeding on the floor.
- Flies.
- Dried faeces behind the sow in lactation.
- Continually used houses without cleaning and disinfection.

Diagnosis

Faeces samples for laboratory examination should be taken from semi-recovered pigs rather than pigs with scour. Diagnosis is best made by submitting a live pig to the laboratory for histological examination of the intestinal wall. *Isospora suis* is the most pathogenic of the three types of coccidia.

Treatment

- ❒ For treatment to be effective it must be given just prior to the invasion of the intestinal wall.
- ❒ Medicate the sow feed with either amprolium premix 1kg/tonne, monensin sodium 100g/tonne (if available) or sulphadimidine 100g/tonne. Feed from the time the sow enters the farrowing house and throughout lactation.
- ❒ Inject each litter with a long-acting sulphonamide at six days of age.
- ❒ Medicate small amounts of milk powder with a coccidiostat such as amprolium or salinomycin and give small amounts daily to the piglets from three days of age onwards.
- ❒ One or two doses of Toltrazuril (Baycox Bayer) at a level of 6.25mg/kg is effective in controlling disease.
- ❒ Depopulating and washing out the pen using a disinfection such as OO-CIDE will remove the coccidial oocysts.

Congenital Tremor (CT) - Shaking Piglets

(Chapter 8 pp264)

This is a sporadic disease seen in newborn pigs. Usually more than one pig is affected in a litter. If the tremors are too great for the piglets to find a teat and suckle then mortality maybe high. Mortality in an affected litter or in a herd outbreak could increase above the norm by 3-10%. The condition decreases as the affected piglets grow.

It would be unusual to find a pig farm that sometime in its history had not experienced one or more litters of trembling piglets. There are 4 possible group causes. The causal virus in group 2, which is by far the commonest cause, is widespread among most if not all pig populations, yet little disease is seen in most herds, presumably because an immunity is established in the sow herd. In new gilt herds however, there can be major outbreaks involving up to 80% of all litters during the first parity. This is an unquantifiable risk in any new gilt herd.

Symptoms

Sows	Piglets
☞ None.	☞ Muscle tremor, only seen when piglets are walk ing around and not when they are asleep.
	☞ Nervous symptoms i.e. shaking of the body.
	☞ Increased mortality in piglets.

Causes / Contributing factors

The causes of the condition are classified into 4 groups based on brain histology.

1. Associated with a classical swine fever.
2. Caused by an unknown virus, possibly a circovirus. Most of the problems in the field are found in this group.
3. Associated with either hereditary disorders seen in the Landrace or Saddleback breeds or with organophosphorus poisoning.
4. Includes aujeszky's disease and Japanese encephalomyelitis virus.

Diagnosis

This is based on clinical evidence although histological examinations in the laboratory can help to differentiate the groups.

Treatment

- ❐ There is no treatment but careful management will greatly reduce mortality.
- ❐ Ensure that piglets are given colostrum at birth and assisted to a teat.
- ❐ Attempts to immunise breeding stock should be carried out.

CRYPTOSPORIDIOSIS

(Chapter 8 pp265)

Cryptosporidia are parasites similar to coccidia that can also cause diarrhoea but at a slightly older age of 8 to 21 days. They can infect people and are also found in other species such as rats and mice.

Symptoms

Sows	Piglets / Weaners
☞ None.	☞ Diarrhoea 8 - 21 days of age.

Causes / Contributing factors

- Rats and mice.
- The main water supplies are sometimes infected.
- Poor hygiene.
- Dirty pens.

Diagnosis

This is made by examining faeces in the laboratory.

Treatment

❒ There is no recognised treatment and the condition is not common.

Cystitis and Pyelonephritis

(Chapter 7 pp203)

Cystitis is inflammation of the bladder and nephritis is inflammation of the kidney. The bacteria causing cystitis are usually *Eubacterium suis* (originally called *Corynebacterium suis*) or sometimes *E. coli*. It is impossible to eradicate these organisms. They are present in every herd.

This disease is an important cause of mortality in all ages of dry sows. Occasionally it may be seen in gilts, even maiden gilts, although this is uncommon unless there has been gross and prolonged faecal contamination of the vulva. In badly affected herds sow mortality can exceed 12% per annum.

Sows die rapidly or respond poorly to treatment remaining chronically diseased. Disease can be so acute that death is the only sign. It is more common in the first 21 days post mating because the urine of the sow becomes alkaline and both *E. suis* and *E. coli* will survive and multiply in alkaline urine.

Reproductive failure is not associated with this disease unless the sow is ill and as a consequence either dies or aborts.

Symptoms

Sows	Piglets
☞ Appear ill.	☞ None. Also uncommon in growing pigs.

- ☞ Not eating.
- ☞ Thin sows.
- ☞ Red rimmed eyes.
- ☞ The area around the vulva is wet and soiled with evidence of blood and pus in the urine.
- ☞ Death.

When cystitis occurs alone:

- ☞ The disease may be prolonged and not fatal.
- ☞ Appetite and the general condition of the sow can be normal.
- ☞ Pus in the urine or a slight discharge clinging to the vulva.
- ☞ This should be distinguished from inflammation of the womb or vagina.

Causes / Contributing factors

- Low water intake.
- Infrequent urination.
- Faulty drinkers.
- Badly drained boar and sow pens increase the risk of infection
- The disease is more common in herds that have high numbers of old sows.
- Squeezing the prepucial sac increases the bacterial load transmitted to the vagina, (which may also result in increased returns to service).
- Sows that are too big for the stalls often adopt a dog sitting position with the vulva becoming heavily contaminated, allowing excessive bacterial multiplication.
- Contamination of the vulva with faeces particularly from weaning to 21 days post mating. This occurs in stalls when solid back boards drop down to the ground level.
- Stress at farrowing can occasionally activate disease.

Diagnosis

By post-mortem examination. Examinations should be carried out on all sows that have died without obvious cause.

In the live animal, diagnosis is based upon clinical signs and evidence of blood and pus in the urine. Urine can be tested for the presence of blood, protein and the pH (acidity or alkalinity) by using paper strip tests. Urine can be collected in clean receptacles, especially if sows are made to stand up 2-3 hours after feeding when they tend to urinate. Affected animals show evidence of blood and protein in the urine and a pH of 7 or more. (Normal urine is slightly acid, that is, less than the pH7.) Sows showing a pH of 8 or more may die in their next pregnancy.

Treatment

- ❒ Lincomycin is effective at a dose level of 10mg/kg. This drug is active against *E. suis*.
- ❒ A more broad spectrum antibiotic however may be required if coliforms or other bacteria are involved. In such cases either ampicillin or amoxycillin at 10 to 15mg/kg should be given daily for 4 to 5 days.
- ❒ On a herd basis, treatment is best carried out using either CTC or OTC at levels of 600g/tonne for a period of 14 days. It may be necessary to repeat this treatment every 4 to 6 weeks.
- ❒ An alternative method is to inject the sow at weaning or at mating with a long-acting single injection of penicillin or amoxycillin.
- ❒ Sows could also be medicated from weaning to 21 days post mating by top dressing with in-feed supplements. The dose used is based on the assumption that the sow will eat 2.5kg of feed per day during this period and the amounts of top dressing should be calculated on the basis of 600g to the tonne of active antibiotic.
- ❒ Antibiotic mastitis tubes or liquid antibiotics can be instilled into the prepuce daily for five days to reduce the weights of infection.

Diarrhoea or Scour

(Chapter 8 pp265)

Of all the diseases in the sucking piglet, diarrhoea is the most common and the most important. In some outbreaks it is responsible for high morbidity and mortality. In a well run herd there should be less than 3% of litters at any one time requiring treatment and piglet mortality from diarrhoea should be less than 0.5%. In severe outbreaks mortality can rise to over 7% and in individual untreated litters up to 100%.

E. coli diarrhoea, clostridial diarrhoea, coccidiosis, TGE and PED all cause diarrhoea in the piglet. *E. coli* is the most important.

At birth the intestinal tract is micro-biologically sterile and it has little immunity to disease producing organisms. Organisms begin to colonise the tract quickly after birth, among them potentially pathogenic strains of *E. coli* and *Clostridium perfringens*. Immunity is initially provided by the high levels of antibodies in colostrum (IgG, IgM, IgA). After the colostral antibodies have been absorbed into the blood stream, the immunity is maintained by the antibody (IgA) which is present in milk. IgA is absorbed into the mucous lining of the intestines. It is essential that the newborn piglet drinks sufficient colostrum soon after birth to prevent potentially pathogenic organisms multiplying against the intestinal wall and causing diarrhoea. It is also essential that the piglet continues to drink milk regularly after the colostrum has gone so that its intestines continue to be lined by protective antibodies.

The antibodies acquired passively from the colostrum and milk are finite and can be overwhelmed by large doses of bacteria present in the environment. The higher the number of organisms taken in, the greater the risk of disease. Environmental stress such as chilling also plays a role because it lowers the piglets resistance. There is thus a delicate balance between the antibody level on the one hand and the weight of infection and stress on the other.

Scour in the piglet can occur at any age during sucking but there are often two peak periods, before 5 days and between 7 and 14 days.

Sudden outbreaks of scour involving large numbers of litters with acute diarrhoea and high mortality suggest TGE, epidemic diarrhoea or PRRS. Rotavirus diarrhoea appears in waves in individual litters or groups of litters and normally in the second half of lactation. Coccidiosis is usually involved in diarrhoea from 7 to 14 days of age. At less than 5 days of age the most common cause is *E. coli* with acute diarrhoea particularly in gilts' litters. Clostridial infections also occur at this age.

Symptoms *(E-Coli)*

Sows

☞ Uncommon.

☞ Usually occur with viral infection.

Piglets

In acute disease:

☞ The only sign may be a previously good pig found dead.

☞ Huddle together shivering or lie in a corner.

☞ The skin around the rectum and tail is wet.

☞ Watery to salad cream consistency scour - distinctive smell.

As the diarrhoea progresses:

☞ Dehydrated.

☞ Sunken eyes.

☞ Leathery skin.

☞ The scour often sticks to the skin of other piglets giving them an orange to white colour.

☞ Prior to death piglets may be found on their sides paddling and frothing at the mouth.

In sub-acute disease:

☞ Signs are similar but the effects on the piglet are less dramatic, more prolonged and mortality tends to be lower.

☞ This type of scour is often seen between 7 to 14 days of age.

☞ Watery to salad cream consistency diarrhoea, often white to yellow in colour.

Causes / Contributing factors

- Poor pen floors.
- Poor pen hygiene associated with bad drainage.
- Poor hygiene procedures, between pens.
- Environmental contamination from one pen to another i.e. boots, brushes, shovels clothing etc.
- Continual use of pens.
- Moisture, warmth, waste food and faeces are ideal for bacterial multiplication.
- Draughts.
- Routine use of milk replacers, particularly if they are allowed

to get stale or contaminated, may increase the incidence.

- Scour is more common in large litters.
- Insufficient colostrum.
    - Poor teat access.
    - Poor crate design.
    - Agalactia in the sow.

Diagnosis

This is based on the clinical examination, the response to treatment (viral diseases do not respond to treatment) and laboratory examination of the scour.

Submit a rectal swab or a recently dead pig or a live pig to the laboratory for cultural examinations and antibiotic sensitivity tests.

Treatment

- ❒ Antibiotics are available for treating scour. Most of these are active against *E. coli* and clostridia.
- ❒ In severe outbreaks of *E. coli* scours the sows feed can be top dressed with the antibiotic daily, from entry into the farrowing house and for up to 14 days post-farrowing to reduce bacterial output in the sows faeces.
- ❒ In light of the history on your farm treat the individual pig or on the first signs of disease treat the whole litter.
- ❒ If a litter is badly scoured dose night and morning for a minimum of two days.
- ❒ Assess the response to treatment. If there is no change within 12 hours then change to another drug as advised by your veterinarian.
- ❒ Always treat piglets less than 7 days of age by mouth.
- ❒ For older pigs where the disease is less acute, injections are equally effective and easier to administer.
- ❒ Provide electrolytes in drinkers. These prevent dehydration and maintain body electrolyte balances.
- ❒ Cover the pen, the creep area and where the pigs defecate with straw, shredded paper, shavings or sawdust.
- ❒ Provide an additional lamp to provide an extra source of heat.
- ❒ If *E. coli* diarrhoea is a problem in litters of younger females it

suggests that immunity levels are low and vaccination should be considered. Inject the gilts twice 2 to 4 weeks apart the second injection at least two weeks before farrowing. These times are variable depending upon the vaccine used. With good management it should not be necessary to vaccinate the sows, only the gilts.

It is not possible to eliminate organisms such as rotavirus, *E. coli* and coccidiosis from the herd and most if not all pigs will be infected with them. Herds can be maintained free of TGE, PED and PRRS. All herds carry clostridia but other factors are required to cause disease.

ECLAMPSIA

(Chapter 8 pp249)

This is an uncommon condition caused by low levels of calcium in the blood stream. It may occur at any stage but is most likely within seven days either side of farrowing. Occasionally seen pre farrowing, normally during lactation.

Symptoms

Sows	Piglets
☞ It is sudden in onset.	☞ N/A
☞ The sow becomes distressed.	
☞ Panting heavily.	
☞ Trembles and shakes.	
☞ Reactive to external stimuli, both touch and sound.	

Causes / Contributing factors

- Loss of calcium in the colostrum.
- Shortage of calcium in the diet.
- Failure of uptake of sufficient calcium.

Diagnosis

This is based on the clinical signs but it can be confused with the porcine stress syndrome (PSS).

Treatment

❒ Give up to 100mls of 40% calcium boroglucinate by injection.

Ideally the injection should be given intravenously but this can be difficult. Alternatively 25mls should be given by intramuscular injection at four separate sites in the neck and rump.

❒ Cool the sow with water.

ELECTROCUTION

(Chapter 8 pp249)

Electrocution of sows and litters occurs sometimes in farrowing houses where electricity is used for heating. Farrowing crates are often connected together throughout the house by various pieces of metal and because of this several animals maybe killed - including piglets.

Symptoms

<u>All Pigs</u>

☞ A variable number of animals are suddenly found dead in one house.

☞ The sows' skin will often be burned where it contacted the metal.

☞ Blood and froth are commonly seen around the nostrils and mouth.

☞ Bones may be fractured.

Causes

- Faulty electricity lines and switches. Trip out switches should be provided in the electricity circuits.
- A common cause however is damage by sows that escape from farrowing crates.

Diagnosis

Post-mortem examinations are necessary to differentiate electrocution from other causes of sudden death. Veterinary certification is usually required for insurance claims.

Note - If you go into your farrowing house and find large numbers of dead animals STOP and THINK ELECTROCUTION or TOXIC GASES.

ENCEPHALOMYOCARDITIS (EMC)

(Chapter 6 pp169)

The main reservoir host for the EMC virus is the rat although mice may also spread it. It infects and causes disease in a wide range of vertebrate animals but pigs appear to be the most susceptible of farm animal species in North America. The virus is worldwide but differs in pathogenicity and virulence in different countries and regions. In most countries of Europe, particularly those in the EU, it tends to be relatively mild or non-pathogenic and disease in pigs is rarely diagnosed.

In Australia the strains appear to be much more virulent for pigs than those in New Zealand. Virulent strains in Florida, the Caribbean and probably Central America damage the heart and cause death whereas those in the Mid West of the US tend to cause reproductive problems.

Clinical disease in pigs tends to occur when rat numbers increase to plague levels.

In affected herds there are usually no clinical signs in weaned and growing pigs.

Symptoms

Sows

In gilts and sows first signs are often :

- ☞ A few abortions near the end of pregnancy.
- ☞ Then over a period of about 3 months the numbers of mummified foetuses and stillbirths increase and pre-weaning mortality rises.
- ☞ The farrowing rate worsens.
- ☞ Affected females may show signs of fever and lack of appetite.

Piglets

- ☞ Poor viable.
- ☞ Usually none.

Causes / Contributing factors

- Pigs can be infected from rats or from rat-contaminated feed or water.
- It does not seem to spread very readily between pigs.

- Incoming breeding stock with pathogenic strain.

Diagnosis

To make a definitive diagnosis the virus has to be isolated and identified or rising antibodies demonstrated in blood samples taken two weeks apart.

EMC could be confused with AD, parvo virus infection and PRRS although there are distinguishing signs between these four. EMCV would be the last on the list of diagnostic priorities in Europe but to a lesser extent in the Mid West USA. Abortion or illness in sows or piglets due to PPV is uncommon and mummified pigs can be examined for the evidence of this infection.

Treatment

❐ There are no methods of treatment.

Endometritis and the Vulval Discharge Syndrome

(Chapter 6 pp180)

A discharge from the vulva post-service does not automatically mean there has been a pregnancy failure, but it will in most cases indicate infection. It is important to record the time when discharges are first seen, their colour and composition and effects on the sow.

Discharges are important between 14-21 days post-service. The lips of the vulva of each sow should be parted daily and any tackiness or small discharge noted. The sow should be marked and if she repeats a problem may be developing. Discharging sows may be pregnant and always pregnancy test before culling.

Discharges in healthy sows are normal up to 5 days post farrowing at mating and 3 - 5 days post mating - only if slight.

Symptoms

<u>Piglets</u>

☞ N/A

<u>Dry Sow</u>

☞ Vulval discharges are common within 3-4 days of farrowing when a thick viscous material may be excreted. This is normal.

☞ If the sow is healthy, the udder is normal and there is no mastitis, ignore it. It is common practice to inject such sows, but this is not necessary under these circumstances.

☞ A heavy smelling bloody discharge may be from a retained piglet or afterbirth.

☞ Endometritis however is important after mating due to ascending infection from the vagina. This results in lost pregnancies or a failure to conceive.

Causes / Contributing factors

Key factors predisposing post service:

- Herds with high numbers of old sows.
- A short lactation length (14-21 days).
- Multiple matings. Cross mating boars.
- Handling the prepuce at mating and squeezing the prepucial sac.
- Matings towards the end of the oestrus period.
- Wet, dirty boar/sow pens. Poor drainage. Continual use.
- Heavy vulval contamination, for example in maiden gilts housed on slats where slurry spills over.
- Re-mating discharging sows.
- Using old boars on young sows.
- Using young boars on older sows.
- Small stalls where the sow adopts a dog sitting position with heavy contamination of the vulva.

Diagnosis

The main organisms associated with endometritis and vulval discharges are opportunist invaders. In some herds no specific organism can be identified, although bacteriological tests may show one or more bacteria predominating either in the prepuce or vagina. A precise diagnosis can be difficult.

Treatment of the boar

❒ You are advised to discuss aspects of treatment with your veterinarian but there are three methods, antibiotics installed into the prepuce, intramuscular injection or by mouth. The latter can be best carried out using in-feed premixes and placing a small amount on the food daily for ten days. The boar could be injected with long-acting antibiotic preparations, but this should be avoided if possible because he can become needle-shy. If leptospirosis is suspected as an initiating factor injections of streptomycin should be given daily for 3 days and this repeated monthly for 5 occasions. Streptomycin is not available in some countries.

Treatment of the sow

- The most effective method is to insert an antibiotic into the anterior vagina up to the cervix (but not actually into it).
- An alternative method of medication is to top dress the feed of the sow from weaning to 21 days post-service. In herds with major problems it may be necessary to medicate all breeding females for a period of ten days with in-feed medication using the appropriate antibiotic.

Enteroviruses (SMEDI)

(Chapter 6 pp169)

These are gut-borne viruses, host specific to the pig, that are included in the group called "SMEDI viruses". SMEDI stands for stillbirth, mummification, embryonic death and infertility. The term is now also commonly used for parvovirus infection. Although these groups of viruses are distinct from that of parvovirus, they are often all grouped together clinically because the signs are similar. The enteroviruses are subdivided into serotypes of which at least 11 are known. Four of these, serotypes 1, 3, 6 and 8, have been implicated in reproductive problems in pigs. Serotype 1 is the Teschen/Talfan virus which can also cause paralysis in pigs. Usually, each pig herd has an array of different serotypes which circulate in weaned and young growing pigs sub-clinically. The pigs are protected by circulatory antibodies derived from their dam's colostrum. By the time they reach breeding age they are solidly immune.

Reproductive problems only occur when a new serotype, to which the gilts are not immune, enters the herd and multiplies in the breeding females. This probably does not happen very often.

It is interesting to note that since the introduction of parvovirus vaccine and the excellent results achieved, the effects from SMEDI viruses would appear to be almost non existent, suggesting that enteroviruses are not important as a cause of reproductive failure.

Symptoms

Sows

- ☞ Embryo mortality.
- ☞ Mummification.
- ☞ Stillbirths.
- ☞ In some cases infertility associated with absorption of embryos also occur.
- ☞ If reproductive failure results there will be increases in embryo mortality, foetal deaths and mummified and stillborn piglets.
- ☞ Infection and disease only occur in non-immune sero-negative animals.
- ☞ Paralysis.

Piglets

- ☞ None.

Causes / Contributing factors

- Ingestion of infected faeces.
- Failure to acclimatise gilts.

Diagnosis

This is carried out by serology and virus isolation. SMEDI can be confused with parvovirus infection and PRRS and occasionally with AD and leptospirosis.

Treatment

- ❐ Treatment is not effective but if a herd experiences problems with enteroviruses in incoming gilts, management practices should ensure that gilts are exposed to infection at least six weeks before breeding. See *chapter 5 pp140* for further information.

Enzootic Pneumonia (EP) - *Mycoplasma Hyopneumoniae* Infection

(Chapter 9 pp308)

Mycoplasma hyopneumoniae causes consolidation of the anterior lobes of the lungs. Clinical signs of enzootic pneumonia only occur in the lactating sow and piglets when the disease has been introduced into a fully susceptible herd for the first time. The breakdown of disease usually takes place over 6 to 8 weeks with sows coming into the farrowing house continuing to be affected.

There is a widely held but erroneous belief that sows and gilts will become carriers and pass this infection to their next litters. They may do so early on and their piglets may cough but by the time they farrow again 4 to 5 months later they will have eliminated the infection and will provide a solid immunity to their piglets via colostrum. If weaning is at 3 to 4 weeks, subsequent litters are not likely to become infected until after weaning.

Symptoms

<u>All pigs</u>

- Coughing.
- Acute pneumonia may develop.
- Severe respiratory embarrassment.
- Sometimes high mortality.

Causes / Contributing factors

- It is commonly transmitted through the movement of carrier pigs.
- Windborne infection for up to 3km (2miles) if the climatic conditions are right.
- Incoming pigs.

Diagnosis

The clinical picture, history of disease and laboratory lung examinations.

Treatment

- Inject all animals at the point of farrowing with long-acting OTC.
- Piglets - give long-acting injections of OTC, tiamulin, lincomycin or tylosin.
- For the treatment of acute pneumonia injections of either lincomycin or tiamulin are advised daily for 4 to 5 days.

Eperythrozoonosis (Epe)

(Chapter 7 pp267)

Eperythrozoonosis is caused by a rickettsial bacterium called *Eperythrozoon suis* (Epe) which attaches itself to the red cells in the blood and damages them resulting in anaemia. Epe can cross the placenta resulting in weak pale pigs at birth. Epe is widespread and can be detected in normal as well as diseased animals. In the majority of herds where it has been identified there have been no clinical problems which casts doubt on the significance of the organism.

Symptoms

Sows

- ☞ Abortion.
- ☞ Agalactia.
- ☞ Anaemia.
- ☞ Fever.
- ☞ Pale skin.
- ☞ Thin sows.
- ☞ Increased repeats.
- ☞ Reduced conception.
- ☞ Reproductive failure.

Piglets

- ☞ In severe cases jaundice may result.
- ☞ Secondary infections tend to occur.
- ☞ More chronic cases result in slow growth and poor-doing pigs.
- ☞ Pale and anaemic pigs.
- ☞ Increased scour.
- ☞ Pneumonia.

Causes / Contributing factors

- ◆ Biting insects.
- ◆ Internal parasites.
- ◆ Lice or mange mites.
- ◆ Cannibalism / Vice (Abnormal behaviour)
- ◆ Sows - method of spread.
  - Vaccinating sows with the same needle
  - Tagging gilts.
  - Feeding back placenta or farrowing house material.
  - Fighting.
  - Vulval and tail biting etc.
- ◆ Piglets - method of spread.
  - Tailing, tooth clipping and iron injections.

Diagnosis

The detection of the organism does not confirm the diagnosis. Identification of the organism in blood smears should be considered to clarify the relationship between Epe and disease. Serological tests have been unreliable but are being improved.

Epe must be differentiated from the following.

- Actinobacillus pleuropneumonia.
- Chronic respiratory disease complexes with PRRS and influenza.
- Glässers disease - *Haemophilus parasuis*.
- Leptospirosis (*L. icterohaemorrhagiae)* .
- Malabsorption and chronic enteritis.
- Pale piglet syndrome - haemorrhages.
- Porcine enteropathy (PE, NE, PHE and PIA).
- Other causes of anaemia (e.g. Iron / copper deficiency).

Treatment

Consider the following treatments and discuss with your veterinarian:

❒ Inject piglets with oxytetracycline at 10mg/kg daily for 4 days or use long-acting preparations, three injections each two days apart.

❒ In-feed medicate sows at 800gms/tonne of OTC for 4 weeks and repeat again 4 weeks later.

❒ Arsanilic acid in-feed at 85gms/tonne is reported to have an effect but in many countries there is no licensed product for food producing animals. Where available it is the drug of choice.

Epitheliogenesis Imperfecta - (Imperfect skin)

(Chapter 10 pp355)

The piglet is born devoid of areas of skin. It usually occurs on legs or flanks.

Symptoms

Sows	Piglets
☞ N/A	☞ Born devoid of areas of skin.

Causes / Contributing factors

- A developmental abnormality.

Diagnosis

This is based on the clinical signs.

Treatment

❒ If the areas are small they will gradually heal but if they are more than 15mm in diameter it will be necessary to infiltrate local anaesthetic, loosen the skin and stitch it together. (See *chapter 15 pp 518* of the main manual). This will depend on the availability of skin and whether the loss is over the flanks where there is plenty of skin, or over the legs where there is little.

❒ In severe cases the piglet should be killed.

ERYSIPELAS

(Chapter 7 pp205)

Swine erysipelas is caused by a bacterium, *Erysipelothrix rhusiopathiae* that is found in most if not all pig farms. Up to 50% of animals may carry it in their tonsils. It is always present in either the pig or in the environment because it is excreted via saliva, faeces or urine. It is also found in many other species, including birds and sheep and can survive outside the pig for a few weeks and longer in light soils. Thus it is impossible to eliminate it from a herd. Infected faeces is probably the main source of infection, particularly in growing and finishing pens.

Disease is relatively uncommon in pigs under 8-12 weeks of age due to protection provided by maternal antibodies from the sow via the colostrum. The most susceptible animals are growing pigs, non vaccinated gilts and up to 4th parity sows.

The organism multiplies in the body, and invades the bloodstream to produce a septicaemia. The rapidity of multiplication and the level of immunity in the pig then determines the clinical symptoms.

Sporadic disease is common in sows but if one sow in a group becomes infected the exposure is high from her urine and faeces and it is advisable to inject all contact animals with penicillin.

Symptoms

These are of three types:

1. Per-acute or acute disease.
2. Sub-acute disease.
3. Chronic disease.

<u>Piglets</u>

☞ Rarely in sucking pigs.

<u>Sows</u>

1. Per-acute or acute disease

☞ The onset is sudden.

- ☞ Often the only sign being death.
- ☞ Death - generalised infection.
- ☞ High temperatures 40°C (108°F).
- ☞ Obviously ill, although others can appear normal.
- ☞ May cause abortion.
- ☞ Mummified piglets.
- ☞ Restricted blood supply causes small raised areas called diamonds in the skin.
- ☞ These are clearly defined become red and finally black, due to dead tissue but no abscesses. Most heal in 7 - 10 days.
- ☞ Often these lumps can be palpated in the early stages before anything can be seen.
- ☞ Stiffness or reluctance to rise indicating joint infection.
- ☞ Sudden death is not uncommon due to an acute septicaemia or heart failure.

2. Sub-acute disease

- ☞ Inappetence.
- ☞ Infertility.
- ☞ Characteristic skin lesions.
- ☞ The temperature ranges from 39-40°C (102-104°F).
- ☞ The disease can be so mild as to be undetected.
- ☞ Some piglets may die in the womb following sub-acute disease and become mummified.

3. Chronic disease

- ☞ This may or may not follow acute, or sub-acute disease.
- ☞ The organism either:
  - Affects the joints producing lameness or
  - The heart valves producing growths.
- ☞ **Boars** infected with erysipelas develop high temperatures and sperm can be affected for the complete development period of 5-6 weeks. Infertility is demonstrated by returns, sows not in pig and poor litter sizes.

Causes / Contributing factors

- ◆ Wet dirty pens.
- ◆ Wet feeding systems, particularly if milk by-products are used,

can become major sources for multiplication of the organism
- Continually populated houses with no all-in and all-out procedures and disinfection.
- Water systems that have become contaminated with the organism.
- Virus infections.
- Feed back of faeces.

Diagnosis

This is determined by the clinical picture and isolation of the organism which is easy to grow in the laboratory. Serology will only indicate exposure to the organism and not necessarily disease. It can only be used to aid diagnosis if rising titres, 14 days apart, are demonstrated and if clinical signs are evident.

Treatment

- ❒ The erysipelas organism is very sensitive to penicillin. Acutely ill animals should be treated with quick acting penicillin twice daily for three days. Alternatively a long-acting penicillin, (check withdrawal periods) given as a single dose to cover 48 hours of treatment, could be given and then repeated.
- ❒ Treat by intramuscular injection 1ml per 10kg (300,000iu/ml).
- ❒ Medicate the feed with 200g/tonne of phenoxymethyl penicillin for 10-14 days. This is a very effective method of prevention, and can be used in major outbreaks of disease. Tetracyclines may also be effective.

Fever

(Chapter 8 pp250)

Fever means a high body temperature of 39-40ºC (103-109ºF). It may occur with little or no other signs or be part of a specific disease.

Symptoms

Dry Sow / (Growing pigs)	Lactating Sow	Piglets
☞ Vomiting.	☞ No milk.	☞ Dull listless.
☞ Temperature.	☞ Temperature.	☞ Not suckling.
☞ Inappetence.	☞ Sow appears dull.	☞ Hair on end.

- ☞ No milk.
- ☞ Dehydration.
- ☞ Increased. respiration.
- ☞ Reddening of skin.

- ☞ Reddening of skin.
- ☞ Mastitis.
- ☞ Metritis.
- ☞ Dehydration.
- ☞ Respiratory rate may be raised.

- ☞ Shivering.
- ☞ Dehydration.

Causes / Contributing factors

- Mastitis or metritis.
- Retention of a dead pig.
- Retention of afterbirth.
- A bacterial septicaemia (e.g. erysipelas).
- Flu or PRRS.
- Secondary bacterial infections associated with flu or PRRS.
- Cystitis/ pyelonephritis.
- Acute stress or eclampsia.
- Heat stroke.

Diagnosis

Check for any of the above conditions. If you cannot find out what the cause is and there are a number of animals involved, veterinary advice should be sought. Bear in mind that depending where in the world your herd is located, fever may be the first clinical sign in such diseases as classical swine fever (hog cholera), African swine fever and aujeszky's disease (pseudorabies).

Treatment

- ❒ In most cases fevers in sows are associated with bacterial infections and a broad spectrum antibiotic should be used. Check the temperature 24 hours after treatment.
- ❒ Broad spectrum antibiotics include, oxytetracycline, trimethoprim/sulpha, amoxycillin and penicillin / streptomycin.

Foot and Mouth Disease (FMD)

This is similar in all pigs see Section 3.

Fractures

(Chapter 7 pp207)

Broken bones are not uncommon in sows and gilts and usually

result from injury and fighting. Spontaneous fractures can occur in bone diseases such as osteochondrosis and osteomalacia, which is associated with calcium phosphorus and vitamins A and D.

Symptoms

<u>All Pigs</u>

- ☞ The onset is always sudden and painful.
- ☞ The sow is reluctant to place any weight on the affected leg or to move.
- ☞ The muscles and tissues over the fracture site are often swollen.
- ☞ Crepitus or the rubbing together of the two broken ends of the bone can often be felt.
- ☞ Fractures of the spinal vertebra are common particularly in the first litter gilt during lactation and after weaning.
- ☞ She usually adopts a dog sitting position and exhibits severe pain on movement.

Causes / Contributing factors

- Bone disease such as osteomalacia, osteoporosis or leg weakness (OCD).
- Low levels of calcium, phosphorus and vitamin D levels in the diet.
- Trauma.
- Fighting.
- Fractures in piglets usually result from the sow.

Diagnosis

This is based upon a history of injury, clinical signs and palpation and it must be differentiated from acute laminitis, arthritis, muscle tearing, bush foot and mycoplasma arthritis.

Treatment

- ❒ Since there is no treatment and movement is painful, the affected pig should be slaughtered or destroyed on the farm.

Frostbite

This is the end result of the destruction of the skin and surface tissues by low temperatures. The ears, tail and feet are particularly vulnerable areas. Frostbite is not uncommon in outdoor pigs.

Symptoms

<u>All Pigs</u>

- ☞ The skin initially becomes pale then bright red, swollen and painful.
- ☞ If exposure to low temperatures continues, the affected tissues die and a line of demarcation develops between damaged and healthy tissues.
- ☞ Secondary skin infections develop.

Causes / Contributing factors

- ◆ Exposure to low temperatures.

Diagnosis

This is based upon skin lesions and a history of exposure to low temperatures. It can be confused with acute infection by erysipelas, salmonella or pasteurella bacteria or a toxic condition.

Treatment

- ❒ Cover affected areas with an antiseptic cream.
- ❒ Topical antibiotic cream may be required to control infections.
- ❒ Move affected animals indoors.

Fungal Poisoning - Mycotoxicosis

(Chapter 13 pp431)

Sometimes when moulds multiply on feeds such as wheat, barley, corn and cotton seed, mycotoxins are produced that can be poisonous. Rations that are suspected of contamination should be examined both for the presence of zearalenone and also other oestrogen like substances.

<u>Zearalenone or F2 Toxin</u> (Fusarium Poisoning)

Symptoms

The clinical signs are distinctive and are dependent up on the levels present in the feed and the state of pregnancy.

- ☞ **Boars** - Semen may be affected with feed levels above 30ppm but not fertility. At higher levels poor libido, oedema of the prepuce and loss of hair may occur.
- ☞ **Gilts (Pre puberty) 1 - 6 months of age** - Swelling and reddening of the vulva and enlargement of the teats and mammary

glands. Rectal and vagina prolapses also may occur in the young growing stock.

- ☞ **Gilts (mature)** - Variable lengths of the oestrus cycle.
- ☞ **Sows** - Anoestrus, which may also be associated with pseudo pregnancy due to the retention of corpus luteum. F2 toxin will not normally cause abortion. If sows are exposed during the period of implantation litter size may be reduced. In lactation piglets may develop enlarged vulva.
- ☞ **Effects on pregnancy** - Complete loss of embryos between implantation and thirty days occurs followed by pseudo pregnancies. Low levels do not appear to affect the mid part of pregnancy, but in the latter stages piglet growth in utero is depressed, with weak splay-legged piglets born. Some of these may have enlarged vulvas.
- ☞ **Effects on lactation** - Low levels have no effect on lactation but the weaning to service interval may be extended.

Causes / Contributing factors

- Mouldy feeds:
  - The purchase of mouldy, damp or badly stored grains.
  - The mixing of contaminated and uncontaminated grains.
  - Holding cereals in moist, damp conditions.
  - Allowing grains to heat.
  - Prolonged usage of feed bins, feed bridging across the bin and development of moulds.
  - Placing compounded feeds into bins whilst they are moist and warm.
  - Poorly maintained bins that allow water to leak in.
  - The bridging of feed in bins over long periods of time and their sudden descent.
  - Prolonged use of automatic feeders and retention of mouldy feed.

Diagnosis

Based on the clinical signs and demonstrating the toxin in feed.

Treatment

- ❒ None is required provided the toxin source is removed. Recycle feed at a 1:10 dilution.

❒ Sows that are in deep anoestrus may respond to injections of prostaglandins or PG 600.

Aflatoxins - (Aspergillus Poisoning)

These toxins are common and their effects are dependent upon the dose and age of the pig. Toxins are found in maize, peanuts and soya beans.

Symptoms

Sows
☞ Abortion.
☞ Agalactia.
☞ Liver damage.
☞ Reduced performance.
☞ Immuno suppression.

Piglets
☞ Unlikely to be any symptoms.

Causes / Contributing factors

- Wet harvests allow fungi to grow.
- Poor storage of feed ingredients.

Diagnosis

Examine feed for evidence of toxin.

Treatment

❒ None.
❒ Remove suspect feed.

Ochratoxin and Citrinin - (Aspergillus & Penicillium Poisoning)

The fungi are found in oats, barley, wheat and maize.

Symptoms

Sows
☞ Liver / kidney damage.
☞ Reduced performance.

Piglets
☞ Unlikely to be any symptoms.

Causes / Contributing factors

- Poor wet harvests allow the fungi to grow.
- Poor storage conditions.

Diagnosis

Clinical and post mortem signs. Toxins identified in feed.

Treatment

❒ None.

- ❒ Remove suspect feeds.
- ❒ Introduce vitamin levels in feed.

Ergotoxins (Ergot poisoning)

These toxins are produced from the fungus ergot found in wheat, oats and rye grass. They interfere with blood flow.

Symptoms

Sow

- ☞ Poor growth.
- ☞ Increased respiration.
- ☞ Depression.
- ☞ Reduced blood supply due to blood vessel contractions.
- ☞ Gangrene at extremities.
- ☞ Tail, ear necrosis.

Piglets

- ☞ Unlikely to be any symptoms.

Causes / Contributing factors

- ◆ Contaminated grains.
- ◆ Poor storage of grains.

Diagnosis

Examine feed for the presence of small black ergot bodies.

Treatment

- ❒ None.
- ❒ Remove affected feed.

Gastric Ulcers

(Chapter 7 pp207)

Erosion and ulceration of the lining of the stomach is a common condition in sows and growing pigs as well. It occurs around the area where the food pipe (oesophagus) enters the stomach. In the early stages of the disease this area becomes roughened and gradually changes as the surface becomes eroded until it is ulcerated. Intermittent bleeding may then take place leading to anaemia or massive haemorrhage may occur resulting in death. The incidence in sows is usually less than 5%.

Symptoms

These depend on the severity of the condition.

Sows

In the less acute form:

- ☞ Pale skin.
- ☞ Weak.
- ☞ Breathless.
- ☞ Diarrhoea.
- ☞ Grinding of the teeth due to stomach pain .
- ☞ Passing of dark faeces containing digested blood.
- ☞ Not eating.
- ☞ Vomiting.
- ☞ A tucked up appearance.

In its most acute form

- ☞ Previously healthy animals are found dead and very pale.

Piglets

- ☞ Uncommon.
- ☞ Often no symptoms.
- ☞ Wasting.

Causes / Contributing factors

There is usually more than one causal factor. They may include nutritional factors, the physical properties of the feed, management deficiencies that lead to stress, and infections.

- Low protein diets.
- Low fibre diets. (The introduction of straw reduces the incidence).
- High energy diets.
- High levels of wheat in excess of 55%.
- Deficiencies of vitamin E or selenium.
- Diets containing high levels of iron, copper or calcium.
- Diets low in zinc.
- Diets with high levels of unsaturated fats.
- Diets based on whey and skimmed milk.
- Pelleting feeds in itself increases the incidence particularly if the meal is too finely ground before pelleting.
- Size of feed particle - the more finely ground the meal the smaller becomes the particle size and the higher the incidence of ulcers. This is still the case if the feed is then pelleted.
- Sometimes there can be problems in changing from pellets to meal.
- Cereals with a high moisture content sometimes seem to con-

tribute to ulcers.

- Excessive aggression between sows.
- Increased stocking densities and movement of pigs.
- Poor management of sows in stalls and tethers.
- Noisy unsympathetic stockmanship in the farrowing rooms.
- Irregular feeding patterns and shortage of feeder space.
- Periods of starvation.
- Poor availability of food or water.
- Transportation.
- Fluctuating environmental temperatures.
- Breed. More common in certain genotypes.
- There is a relationship between outbreaks of pneumonia and the incidence of gastric ulceration.
- Ulceration may occur following bacterial septicaemias such as those associated with erysipelas and swine fever.

Diagnosis

This can be made on the clinical signs and post mortem lesions in sows which die. A faeces sample can be examined for the presence of blood and to eliminate parasites.

Gastric ulcers can be confused for the massive intestinal bleeding and anaemia that occurs in bloody gut (PE) but this is usually confined to gilts. Anaemia can also be associated with eperythrozoonosis, the stomach worm *Hyostrongylus rubidus*, chronic mange and nutritional deficiencies.

Treatment

- ❐ Move the affected animal from its existing housing into a loose bedded peaceful environment.
- ❐ Feed a weaner type diet containing highly digestible materials.
- ❐ Inject multi vitamins, particularly vitamin E together with 0.5 to 1g of iron intramuscularly and repeat on a weekly basis.
- ❐ Add an extra 100g vitamin E / tonne to the diet for two months and assess the results.
- ❐ Change staff around.
- ❐ Check all the factors listed above that contribute to ulcers particularly the particle size.

GLÄSSERS DISEASE (*HAEMOPHILUS PARASUIS* HPS)

(Chapter 7 pp269)

This is caused by the bacterium *Haemophilus parasuis (Hps)*, of which there are at least fifteen different types. It is found throughout the world and organisms are present even in high health herds. If such herds are set up using SPF or MEW techniques and are free from Hps it can be devastating when they first become contaminated, producing an anthrax-like disease with high mortality in sows. In the majority of herds in which the bacterium is endemic, sows produce a strong maternal immunity which normally persists in their offspring until 8 to 12 weeks of age. As a result, the effects of the infection in weaners are usually nil or minimal. The pigs become sub-clinically infected when still protected and then stimulate their own immune response. If however the maternal immunity wears off before they become infected they may develop severe disease. It can also act as a secondary pathogen to other major diseases particularly enzootic pneumonia (EP) (*Mycoplasma hyopneumoniae*). Outbreaks of disease are sometimes experienced in sucking pigs, particularly in gilt herds.

Hps attacks the smooth surfaces of the joints, coverings of the intestine, lungs, heart and brain causing pneumonia, heart sac infection, peritonitis and pleurisy. It is respiratory spread.

Symptoms

Sows

☞ Rare disease in the dry sow unless naive.

Occasionally seen in gilts:

☞ Lameness / stiffness.

☞ Slight swellings over the joints and tendons.

☞ Meningitis rarely.

Piglets

Acute disease:

☞ Rapidly depressed.

☞ Elevated temperature.

☞ Inappetence .

- ☞ Reluctant to rise.
- ☞ Characteristic feature a short cough of 2-3 episodes.
- ☞ Sudden death in good sucking piglets is not uncommon.
- ☞ Also causes individual cases of arthritis and lameness with fever and inappetence.

Chronic disease:

- ☞ Pale and poor growing pigs.
- ☞ Sudden deaths may occur.

Causes / Contributing factors

- ◆ Respiratory spread. Disease may be precipitated by PRRS, Flu or EP.
- ◆ Poor environments, draughts etc. predispose.
- ◆ Stress.

Diagnosis

This is made by clinical observations, post-mortem examinations and isolation of the organism in the laboratory. Glässers disease has to be differentiated from actinobacillus suis infection, App, mulberry heart disease, streptococcal meningitis and arthritis and bacterial septicaemias.

Treatment

- ❒ Hps has a wide antibiotic sensitivity including amoxycillin, ampicillin, OTC, sulphonamides, penicillin and ceftiofur.
- ❒ Treatment must be given early, particularly if cases of meningitis are occurring.
- ❒ Treat for 2 to 3 days.
- ❒ Identify when the onset of disease is likely to occur and inject 3 to 4 days prior to this to prevent disease, with long-acting penicillin.
- ❒ Medicate the water with amoxycillin or phenoxymethyl penicillin for 4-5 days over the period of risk.

Greasy Pig Disease - (Exudative Epidermitis)

(Chapter 7 pp270)

This is caused by the bacterium *Staphylococcus hyicus* which lives normally on the skin without causing disease. It is not known why sometimes it flares up and causes a dermatitis which oozes slippery fluid. It produces toxins which are absorbed into the system and damage the liver and kidneys. In the sucking piglet disease is usually confined to individual animals, but it can be a major problem in new gilt herds and weaned pigs. During the days immediately preceding farrowing the bacterium multiples profusely in the sow's vagina so that piglets are infected during the birth process or soon after.

Symptoms

Sows

☞ Uncommon.

Piglets

☞ Severely affected piglets will die.
☞ Localised lesions on the flanks and behind ears. Lesions usually commence with small, dark, localised areas of infection around the face or on the legs.
☞ The skin along the flanks the belly and between the legs changes to a brown colour gradually involving the whole of the body.
☞ The skin becomes wrinkled with flaking of large areas and it has a greasy feel.
☞ In severe cases the skin turns black and the piglets die.
☞ A more localised picture is seen if the sow has passed some immunity to the piglet, with small circumscribed lesions approximately 5-10mm in diameter that do not spread.

Causes / Contributing factors

- One possibility may be that the sharp eye teeth inject it into the cheeks during competition for a teat.
- Abrasions on the knees from sucking may also trigger it off.
- Abrasions from poor concrete surfaces or metal floors, side panels and damaged metal feeding troughs.
- Faulty procedures for iron injections, removing tails and teeth.
- Abnormal behaviour.
- Fighting and skin trauma at weaning.

Diagnosis

This is based on the characteristic skin lesions. It is important to culture the organism and carry out an antibiotic sensitivity test. A moist wet area should be identified, the overlying scab removed and a swab rubbed well into the infected area.

Treatment

❒ Inject affected piglets daily for 5 days, or on alternate days with a long-acting antibiotic to which the organism is sensitive.

❒ Antibiotics include amoxycillin, OTC, ceftiofur, cephalexin, gentamycin, lincomycin or penicillin.

❒ Topical application of antibiotics can also be of use. Novobiocin, an antibiotic used for treating mastitis in dairy cows, can be mixed with mineral oil and sprayed onto the skin or the piglets dipped into a solution of it.

❒ Piglets become very dehydrated and should be offered electrolytes by mouth.

❒ Long-acting injections can be given 2 to 3 days before the first signs are likely to appear as a method of prevention. Use either long-acting amoxycillin or OTC if indicated.

❒ In severe outbreaks an autogenous vaccine can be prepared from the organism and sows injected twice 4 and 2 weeks prior to farrowing to raise immunity in the colostrum.

❒ If the problem is occurring in gilt litters, cross suckling these piglets, using older sows at birth, for 4 or 5 hours can be of value.

HAEMATOMA

(Chapter 9 pp317)

A haematoma is a pocket of blood that forms beneath the skin or in muscle tissue and usually results from ruptured blood vessels following trauma particularly over the shoulders, flanks or the hind quarters. Often the ear of the sow may be damaged from rubbing due to mange or fighting.

Symptoms

Sows

☞ Blood from the vulva.

☞ Head on one side.

☞ Large swellings which develop suddenly.

Piglets

☞ Uncommon but as for sow.

☞ The swellings contain blood or serum.

Causes / Contributing factors

- Fighting.
- Mange.
- Trauma.

Diagnosis

This is based on the clinical signs. Differentiate from an abscess, test with a needle and syringe

Treatment

❒ In most cases these will resolve over two to three weeks once sufficient pressure has built up in the tissues the haemorrhage stops and a clot is formed which is gradually removed by the normal body repair mechanisms.

❒ In some cases the haematoma may become infected and an abscess develops. This should be dealt with as described under abscess.

❒ It is inadvisable in the sow to lance a haematoma if it has not developed into an abscess. Sample the fluid first by syringe and needle. If blood is withdrawn the haematoma is of recent origin and if serum is present it is long standing. Leave both alone.

❒ Animals with a large haematoma of the ear are best culled.

Heat Stroke

This usually occurs where ventilation has failed or in extremely hot weather.

Symptoms

Sows

☞ Distress.

☞ A very high respiratory rate.

☞ Muscle trembling.

☞ Weakness.

☞ Prostration.

☞ Vomiting.

☞ Diarrhoea may be seen.

☞ Rectal temperature may rise to 43°C (109°F)

Piglets

☞ Uncommon, but as for sow.

Causes / Contributing factors

- High temperatures.
- Exposure to sunlight.
- Combined with high humidity and poor ventilation in indoor housing.

Diagnosis

The history and clinical signs.

Treatment

- ❒ Give immediate treatment.
- ❒ Immerse the animal in cold water or spray.
- ❒ Dribble cold water into the rectum using a flutter valve.

HYPOGLYCAEMIA - LOW BLOOD SUGAR LEVEL

(Chapter 7 pp271)

During the first few days of life the newborn piglet is unable to mobilise the low glycogen reserves in the liver to provide adequate levels of glucose in the blood. It is therefore dependent for energy on a regular intake of lactose from the sows milk. If a piglet cannot obtain sufficient lactose to maintain its energy output, it runs out of energy, its body temperature drops and ultimately it goes into a coma and dies.

Hypoglycaemia usually occurs in the first 12-24 hours of birth.

Symptoms

<u>Sows</u>

- ☞ N/A

<u>Piglets</u>

- ☞ Laid on belly.
- ☞ Shivering.
- ☞ Becoming very cold.
- ☞ Paddling.
- ☞ Frothing at the mouth.
- ☞ Comatosed.
- ☞ Eyes are sunken and the head bent backwards.

Causes / Contributing factors

- Low level of sugar in the blood.
- No milk - starvation.

- Severe chilling.
- Wet pens.
- Low viable piglets.

Diagnosis

This is based on the clinical signs. Examine the eyes to see that there is no evidence of rapid back and fore lateral movements which would indicate meningitis not hypoglycaemia.

Treatment

- ❒ The condition must be recognised early if treatment is to be successful.
- ❒ Immediately remove the piglet to a warm draught free environment at 30°C (86°F).
- ❒ Feed the piglet with sow's or alternatively cow's colostrum or 20% dextrose solution by syringe or stomach tube every 20 minutes until it has returned to normal. Then introduce the piglet to a newly farrowed sow.
- ❒ Identify potential hypoglycaemic piglets at birth and treat as described under poor viable piglets.

Jaw and Snout Deviation

(Chapter 7 pp209)

This is a common yet little recognised condition in the sow. When the jaw is at rest, a proportion of sows (often around 5%) and particularly those housed in confinement, show a misalignment of the lower jaw to the left or right of centre. In extreme cases this can give the appearance of rhinitis but it is of no significance.

Symptoms

Sows
- ☞ Misalignment of the lower jaw when at rest.
- ☞ The upper jaw and nose become shortened and flattened, in some cases to a grotesque degree.

Piglets
- ☞ N/A

Causes / Contributing factors

- Constant trauma from bar biting or the use of nipple drinkers.
- Infection of the bone as a result of faulty teeth clipping.
- Prolonged feeding of very finely ground meal in narrow troughs.

Diagnosis

This is based on the clinical symptoms and absence of rhinitis.

Treatment

❐ None. The condition is of no consequence.

LAMENESS

(Chapter 7 pp209)

Lameness is a common cause for culling sows second only to reproductive failure. Cases can occur at any time during the dry period or in lactation. Increased unplanned culling for lameness increases the non productive sow days so reducing the litters per sow per year. Often problems involve first parity or second parity animals before they have reached the most productive part of their life. Sows culled for severe lameness have to be shot on the farm because they should not be transported.

To investigate a lameness problem it is helpful to have accurate records on each sow which should include the following:

- Sow number.
- Breed or genetic line.
- Parity and age.
- Date of mating.
- Date of farrowing.
- Date of weaning.
- Date of lameness.
- Type of lameness.
- Housing area.

Alternatively you could use the farrowing rate loss sheet that is used in the dry period.

Symptoms

Sows

☞ Pig off food.
☞ Sometimes fever.
☞ Reluctance to stand.
☞ Swollen joints.
☞ Evidence of other diseases.

Piglets

☞ As for sows.
☞ Shivering.

- Loss of balance.
- Arthritis.

Causes / Contributing factors

Causes of lameness in breeding animals can be separated into infectious and non infectious.

The common ones* are listed below.

Infectious causes

- Erysipelas *
- Foot rot, Bush foot *
- Glässers disease in gilts.
- Haemophilus arthritis.
- Mycoplasma arthritis.
- Salmonella arthritis.
- Streptococcal arthritis.

Non infectious causes

- Damage to nerves.
- Fractures.
- Haematomas.
- Laminitis (inflammation of the tissues attaching to the hoof).
- Leg weakness (OCD).
- Myositis (inflammation of muscles).
- Nutritional deficiencies.
- Osteitis (inflammation of bone).
- Osteochondrosis (degeneration of bone growth plate and cartilage).
- Osteomalacia (softening of bone, calcium and phosphorus deficiency).
- Osteomyelitis (inflammation of bone and bone marrow).
- Osteoporosis (weak bones, imbalance of calcium and phosphorus).
- Penetrated sole.
- Periostitis (inflammation of the membrane around bone).
- Separation of the muscle from the pelvis.
- Separation of the head of the femur.
- Split horn (poor hoof quality).
- Torn muscle and/or ligament.
- Trauma.

Diagnosis

This is based on the clinical signs.

Treatment

- ❒ Specific treatment will depend on the cause.
- ❒ Give antibiotics such as oxytetracycline or amoxycillin by injection daily for 3 - 4 days.

LAMINITIS

(Chapter 7 pp211)

Inflammation of the soft highly vascular sensitive tissues that connect the bone to the hoof. It is an uncommon but very painful condition causing animals to walk on their knees.

Symptoms

Sows

- ☞ Animals walking on their knees.
- ☞ Lameness.
- ☞ Pain over hooves.

Piglets

- ☞ N/A

Causes / Contributing factors

- ◆ The cause is unknown.

Diagnosis

This is based on the clinical signs.

Treatment

- ❒ Affected pigs should be destroyed.
- ❒ Cortisone injections in non pregnant animals in mild cases.

LEG WEAKNESS - OSTEOCHONDROSIS (OCD)

(Chapter 7 pp211)

"Leg weakness" is an imprecise term used to describe different forms of lameness. For example, it is sometimes used to describe poor leg conformation. More often it is used to describe a clinical condition associated with degeneration of the bone and cartilage, called osteochondrosis (OCD).

Changes in the cartilage that lead to clinical OCD take place in most modern pigs from as early as two months of age. The severity and its effect depend largely on the environment and the speed of growth of the animal. OCD in modern pigs results from the many years of selecting animals for rapid growth, large muscle mass, and efficient feed conversion and therefore much greater weight on the growth plates whilst they are still immature, together with the stresses of intensive methods of production.

OCD may be seen within three months of gilts being introduced on to the farm, during their first pregnancy, in lactation or in the first 2 to 3 weeks post weaning.

Symptoms

Piglets

- None.

Sows

In acute cases of OCD:

- There is separation of the bones at the growth plate resulting from sudden movement.
- The animal walks on three legs, the affected leg swinging freely.
- Crepitus, the rubbing of the broken bones together, can usually be felt.
- Fractures in the spine can also occur particularly during lactation and immediately post weaning.
- In such cases the sow is in acute pain.
- Often in a dog sitting position with the hind legs well forward.

In chronic cases of OCD, the onset is gradual.

- The sow shows abnormal leg conformation and gait with or without stiffness and pain.
- The temperature and affected joints remain normal.
- The front legs may be straight, the pig walking with a long step on its toes, or the knees may be bent inwards or flexed, the pig walking with short steps. In some old sows, the pasterns may be dropped. The feet may be rotated or twisted.
- The hind legs are often straight, the pig walking with a swinging action from the hips. In some cases the legs are tucked beneath the body. The hocks are turned inwards and are close

together. The pig walks with a goose stepping action. Again in old sows the pasterns may be dropped.

Causes / Contributing factors

- Environmental factors that cause the foot to slip on the floor.
- The design of slats can contribute to OCD. Some slats slope to the edges from the centre and are so smooth that when the animals stand, the feet slip into the gaps, causing repeated pressure on the growth plates.
- Full confinement of pregnant gilts when they are still growing can be a major contributing factor.
- Are the gilts mixed with sows at weaning? The modern hybrid gilt often suckles produces large litters and large amounts of milk which depletes her body calcium and phosphorous. The bones become weak and are therefore more prone to injury.
- High levels of vitamin A (in excess of 20,000 iu/kg) particularly in the younger growing pigs can interfere with the normal development of the growth plates.
- High stocking densities increase the incidence, particularly in the growing period and where animals are housed on solid concrete floors or slats.
- Trauma.

Diagnosis

This is based on the clinical signs. There are no laboratory tests and post-mortem examinations may be misleading because many pigs that were not lame before death may be found to have lesions.

OCD has to be distinguished from *Mycoplasma hyosynoviae* and erysipelas arthritis.

Treatment

- ❒ There is no specific treatment for OCD, however, at an early stage the sow should be moved from its existing environment to a well-bedded pen where the foot can grip. If not, the lesions progress and ultimately arthritis and permanent lameness develop.
- ❒ In acute cases of OCD the sows should be culled immediately.

LEPTOSPIROSIS

(Chapter 6 pp186)

Leptospira are long slender spiral-shaped bacteria, found in most mammalian host species. Over 160 serotypes are known, generally called serovars, with cross infections occurring between some host species. Each serotype has one or more (usually only two or three) reservoir hosts which multiply it up and maintain it. A serotype can remain as a life-long infection in its reservoir host.

The pig is a reservoir host for *Leptospira pomona*, *L. tarassovi*, *L. bratislava* and *L. muenchen*, the last two being very closely related. It is not a reservoir host for *L. icterohaemorrhagiae* but it can be infected from rats urine and become ill. It can also become infected by other serotypes from other animals urine, for example *L. canicola* from dogs and *L. hardjo* from cattle but the infections are subclinical and do not result in disease. The pig is then an incidental host i.e. does not perpetuate the infection and is only responsible for minimal spread.

L. pomona causes important reproductive problems in female breeding pigs spreading slowly through the herd. It remains in the herd permanently unless steps are taken to eradicate it. It is not in the UK or Ireland and seems to have disappeared from Western Europe but is widespread throughout the rest of the pig rearing world. In America the skunk is an alternative reservoir host.

L. tarassovi causes a similar syndrome (i.e. a collection of signs and lesions) to *L. pomona* but tends to be milder and to spread more slowly. It is found in Eastern Europe and the Antipodes. It is thought that some wild animals are also reservoir hosts.

The pig is also a reservoir host for certain subtypes of *L. bratislava* and *L. muenchen* which are widespread throughout the pigs of the world. They cause a different syndrome to *L. pomona* and *L. tarassovi* and affect mainly pregnant gilts and second litter females because they will not previously have encountered it.

Once these organisms are introduced into a herd the pigs become permanent carriers with infection of the kidneys and intermittent excretion of the organism into the urine. *L. bratislava/muenchen* also permanently inhabit the fallopian tube of sows and the reproductive organs of boars and they are spread in semen.

Disease is uncommon in the sucking pig and would only infect individuals.

Remember that this disease can be transmitted to people.

Symptoms

Sows

In acute outbreaks:

- ☞ Inappetence.
- ☞ Fever.
- ☞ Depression may be observed.

Chronic low grade disease is more common with:

- ☞ Abortions.
- ☞ Stillbirths.
- ☞ Increase in poor, non-viable pigs.

Piglets

- ☞ Uncommon.
- ☞ Illness.
- ☞ Inappetence.
- ☞ Jaundice.
- ☞ Blood in urine.
- ☞ Severely infected pigs die.

If abortions in a herd are more than 1% then investigations for leptospirosis should be considered. A reduction in farrowing rates and numbers of live pigs born per sow is also an associated factor particularly with *L. bratislava* infection.

Signs associated with acute *L. bratislava* disease:

- ☞ Repeat breeders are common particularly in first and to some extent second pregnancy gilts.
- ☞ This often follows embryo loss and there may be copious vaginal discharges.
- ☞ Late term abortions.
- ☞ An increase in premature piglets.
- ☞ An increase in stillbirths.
- ☞ Mixed litters of live poor pigs and dead piglets at birth.
- ☞ An increase in mummified pigs.
- ☞ An increase in repeat breeding animals.
- ☞ Often there is a two year cycle of disease.
- ☞ Reproductive failure occurs in second litter females, rather than gilts following their introduction to older carrier boars.
- ☞ Disease is less common in older animals.

☞ In long standing carrier herds disease can be difficult to recognise.

Causes / Contributing factors

Infection can enter the herd in one of three ways:

1. Introduction of infected gilts and boars.
2. Infection brought into the herd by other animals; rats, mice and dogs can be reservoirs of infection.
3. Exposure of the herd to indirect sources of contamination, e.g.: contaminated water, poor floor surfaces allow urine to pool. Spread in urine.

Diagnosis

This is difficult but the following will help:

- Records. Study the levels of abortions, repeats, stillbirths, week piglets and the age of occurrence in sows and gilts.
- Study the clinical picture.
- Blood sample suspicious animals and repeat 2-3 weeks later. Look for rising antibody titres e.g. 1st sample result 1:100, 2nd result 1:800. This would confirm active infection and indicate probable involvement.
- Blood sample ten females that have a history of infertility.
- In chronic disease however, the significance of titre levels are very difficult to assess.
- Test the aborted foetuses, urine or kidneys and fallopian tubes of slaughtered gilts.
- Eliminate other diseases - Chronic PRRS, endometritis.
- Eliminate non infectious causes of infertility - Summer infertility, management failures.
- The symptoms of leptospirosis can be mistaken for other causes of infertility.

Treatment

❐ Medicate the feed with tetracyclines, either oxytetracycline or chlortetracycline at levels of 800g/tonne. Feed for a period of three weeks followed by a further course six weeks later, and repeat this for four treatment periods.

❐ An initial three week course of 800g of tetracycline followed by a further eight week course at 400g.

- ❒ Strategic medication. Where there is a history of periodic infertility, in-feed medication can be targeted just prior to the expected time of disease.
- ❒ Inject sows at weaning time with streptomycin if available at 25mg/kg. Boars should be treated with this drug once every six weeks. Alternatively semi-synthetic penicillins could be used.
- ❒ Introduce antibiotic into the anterior vagina post-service. This is the same procedure to that described under vaginal discharges, and involves the use of an AI catheter and the deposition of antibiotic into the anterior vagina 6-18 hours after the last mating. Ampicillin, amoxycillin, or penicillin/dihydrostreptomycin could be used. *(Chapter 15 pp 474)*. Discuss with your veterinarian.

Listeriosis

This is caused by the bacterium *Listeria monocytogenes* which may colonise the tonsils and be passed out in faeces. Listeria are wide spread in nature and are often found in cheese and silage. Exposure results in infection but disease is uncommon.

Symptoms

Sows	Piglets
☞ None.	☞ The bacterium may cause a septicaemia in piglets.
	☞ Nervous signs possibly meningitis.
	☞ Weak piglets at birth.
	☞ Pneumonia.

Causes / Contributing factors

- Stress causing the bacteria to invade the system.
- PRRS or Flu.
- Heavy environmental exposure

Diagnosis

Laboratory examinations are necessary.

Treatment

- ❒ Listeria are usually sensitive to penicillin and ampicillin.
- ❒ In outbreaks it is necessary to identify the sources of infection and reduce the exposure to them.

Mange Mites (*Sarcoptes Scabiei*)

(Chapter 11 pp385)

Mange is a parasitic disease of the skin caused by one of two mites either *Sarcoptes scabiei* or *Demodex phylloides.* Sarcoptic mange (sometimes called scabies) is by far the most common and important because it is irritant and uncomfortable for the pig, causing it to rub and damage the skin which becomes unsightly. It significantly depresses growth rate and feed efficiency. The life cycle is direct and takes 14-15 days from adult to adult to complete. The mite dies out quickly away from the pig, under most farm conditions, in less than five days. This is an important factor in control. If a herd is free from mange, it is one of the easiest of diseases to keep out because it can only be introduced by carrier pigs. However, once it is introduced it tends to become permanently endemic unless control measures are taken.

Symptoms

Piglets

- ☞ Skin irritation after 7 days.

Sows

In acute disease:

- ☞ Ear shaking .
- ☞ Severe rubbing of the skin against the sides of the pen. Approximately three to eight weeks after initial infection the skin may become sensitised to the mite protein. A severe allergy may develop in some pigs with very tiny red pimples covering the whole of the skin.
- ☞ Intense irritation and rubbing to the point where bleeding may occur.

In chronic disease:

- ☞ Thick asbestos-like lesions on the ear, along the sides of the neck, the elbows, the front parts of the hocks and along the top of the neck.

Causes / Contributing factors

- The mite spreads directly from pig to pig, either by close skin contact or contact with recently contaminated surfaces.

- The boar helps to maintain infection in the herd because he is constantly in direct skin contact with breeding females and he remains a chronic carrier.
- If pigs are housed in groups there is increased opportunity for spread.
- Newly purchased pigs.
- Disease is more easily spread where sows are group housed.
- Continually housed pens.

Diagnosis

This is confirmed by demonstrating the presence of the mite. Scrapings are taken from suspicious lesions on the skin and particularly inside the ears. A teaspoon is an ideal instrument to scarify material from the interior of the ear. This material can be spread onto a piece of black paper and left for ten minutes. Mange mites which are rounded in shape and only 0.5mm in length may be just visible to the naked eye. However to positively identify the mite the scrapings should be submitted to a laboratory for microscopic examination. An ELISA blood test is also available.

Treatment

Mange is an expensive disease not only because of its economic effects on the pig but also the costs and necessity for repeated treatment.

- ❐ **Adult stock** - Examine the breeding herd for the presence of chronic lesions. Identify such animals for special treatment. These chronic lesions, found especially in the ears behind the elbow and on the legs, can be difficult to eradicate and they remain a constant source of infection.

  If they are evident in the ears dress them three times, once every 10 days with either 1ml of phosmet or spray with 1% benzyl benzoate. If they are on the skin scrub with amitraz every 10 days.
- ❐ Treat all the breeding herd (gilts, sows and boars) with phosmet 20% 1ml to 10kg weight on one day. Repeat this 10-14 days later. Alternatively use ivermectin or doramectin by injection or ivermectin in feed every 4 - 6 months.
- ❐ **Weaners** - Treat pigs on the day of weaning with 0.75 - 1ml of

phosmet using a pump applicator or give an ivermectin injection. Alternatively either medicate the creep feed with ivermectin for 7 days or the water for the first five days of weaning. The latter is best carried out using a water tank with a water bowl attached. The total weight of weaned pigs is calculated and the required daily ivermectin dose added to sufficient water that will be consumed in 24 hours. The water in the tank is agitated three times daily. The water is freshly medicated each day. Ivermectin as a sheep drench has been used successfully for this purpose at a dose level of 12.5ml/100kg liveweight. Discuss with your veterinarian.

- ❐ Treated pigs should only be moved into **cleaned washed pens** that have been sprayed with a parasecticide such as amitraz and left empty for at least three days, preferably five to six.
- ❐ If mange is active at the onset in the growing herd medicate with ivermectin in-feed for seven days.

Mastitis - Inflammation of the Mammary Glands

(Chapter 8 pp237)

Mastitis in one or more mammary glands is caused by a variety of bacteria or it may be secondary to other diseases. It is a common condition that occurs sporadically in individual sows or sometimes as herd outbreaks. It starts around farrowing and becomes clinically evident up to 12 hours later. It can arise because bacteria have gained entry to one or more mammary glands for the first time, or it may be a flare-up of a long-standing sub-clinical latent infection. The route of entry of the bacteria is probably the teat orifice but it may be from the blood stream or by injection on piglets' teeth. It also commonly occurs at weaning time.

The bacteria that cause mastitis in the sow can be grouped into three broad categories: coliform bacteria, staphylococci and streptococci, and miscellaneous bacteria.

Coliform mastitis - Coliform bacteria are related to *E. coli*, the commonest being *E. coli* itself and klebsiella. They produce a severe acute mastitis which results in reduced milk yield, a very ill sow and poor "doing" piglets. Marked discoloration of the skin over the udder and dark blueing of surrounding skin, ears and tail is a feature.

Herd problems can develop because the organisms are present in faeces and may also be in sows' urine. Consequently, they may be everywhere in a piggery. Coliform mastitis may thus be regarded as environmental in origin.

Staphylococcal and streptococcal mastitis - These are usually less acute and less severe than coliform mastitis. They tend to occur sporadically in individual sows in one or more glands and usually do not make the sow ill. The exception is an acute severe staphylococcal infection usually in a single gland which becomes swollen, hard and discoloured and makes the sow toxic.

Unlike coliform bacteria the source of these organisms is not usually the contaminated environment but the skin and possibly orifices of the sow herself. There is some evidence to suggest that as in the dairy cow and sheep some of these bacteria may persist sub-clinically in the udder and then flare up at or after farrowing

Miscellaneous bacteria - These include organisms such as pseudomonas which can produce a serious mastitis and toxaemia and which are often resistant to antibiotic treatment. Fortunately such infections are rare.

Symptoms

<u>Sows</u>

Acute disease

☞ Inappetence at farrowing or before if mastitis is already developing.

☞ Obviously ill will not suckle.

☞ Fever.

☞ Mucous membrane of her eyes are brick red.

☞ Affected glands swollen, red colour and painful.

☞ Discoloration of the ears and the whole of the udder, but particularly over the affected glands.

Chronic disease (Usually seen in dry sows):

<u>Piglets</u>

☞ Hungry.

☞ Thin.

☞ Squealing due to lack of milk.

- ☞ Mammary tissue is infiltrated with hard lumps that are usually not painful when palpated.
- ☞ They may ulcerate to the surface and become a potential source of infection to other sows.

Causes / Contributing factors

- The continual use of farrowing houses.
- Poor farrowing pen hygiene, bad drainage, inadequate and poor quality bedding.
- The use of saw dust or shavings for bedding that become soaked in water or urine.
- A warm temperature for the organisms to multiply.
- Worn pitted farrowing house floors.
- Wet farrowing house floors.
- Contaminated drinking water.
- Adverse temperatures, draughts and poor ventilation in the farrowing houses.
- A build up of faeces behind the sows.
- Klebsiella in the water system.

Diagnosis

The clinical signs are usually sufficient to diagnose mastitis. However if there is a herd problem with a number of sows affected, you should examine all animals clinically at farrowing and again at weaning, to determine the starting point of the mastitis. A sample of the secretions from the infected quarters should be submitted to a laboratory for examination. This is carried out by wiping the teat end with cotton wool soaked in surgical spirit, injecting the sow with 0.5ml of oxytocin and once there is a good flow squirt the milk on to a sterile swab. The swab should be immersed in a transport medium. It is very important that mastitis is diagnosed early and that prompt treatment is given.

Treatment

- ❒ Oxytocin to let milk down (0.5ml).
- ❒ The following antibiotics could be used: OTC, penicillin and streptomycin, trimethoprim/sulpha, semi-synthetic penicillins such as amoxycillin, framycetin, tylosin, enrofloxacin and ceftiofur.

- ❒ In very severe cases the sow should be injected twice daily.
- ❒ Corticosteroids or flunixin may also be prescribed by your veterinarian.
- ❒ In severe outbreaks the sow can be injected 12 hours prior to farrowing with an appropriate long-acting injection.
- ❒ The udder can be sprayed daily for 2 days with an iodine based dairy teat dip, commencing 24 hours before farrowing is due to start.

MENINGITIS

(Chapter 9 pp336)

Meningitis is uncommon in the sow but it is sometimes secondary to middle ear infection. If an infectious disease enters a herd for the first time sporadic cases in sows may be seen. Meningitis is seen in the sucking pigs and weaners associated with streptococcal infections. See Streptocal meningitis.

Symptoms

Sows

- ☞ The sow is off feed.
- ☞ Trembling with an unsteady gate.
- ☞ The temperature is elevated, often as high as 42°C (108°F).

As the meningitis develops:

- ☞ The eye moves sideways.
- ☞ Fits occur and the sow cannot stand.
- ☞ The head may be on one side.

Piglets / Weaners

- ☞ Shivering.
- ☞ Lateral movement of eyes (nystagmus).
- ☞ Fits.
- ☞ On side paddling.

Causes / Contributing factors

- ◆ Middle ear infection.
- ◆ Specific bacteria e.g. streptococci, *Haemophilus parasuis.*
- ◆ Aujeszky's disease.
- ◆ Poisons.
- ◆ Poor environments in nurseries.

Diagnosis

This is based upon the signs in an individual sow, or if there are a number of cases, a specific infectious disease. It may require a post-mortem examination, including histology of the brain and culture of the causal organism to confirm the diagnosis.

Meningitis must be differentiated from the following.

Acute kidney infection.

Aujeszky's disease (AD) (PR).

Brain abscess.

Heat stroke.

Middle ear infection.

Poisons.

Water deprivation (salt poisoning).

Treatment

- ❐ Treatment depends upon the cause. Always consider the common ones first in sows which include middle ear infection, brain abscess, water deprivation and in some countries aujeszky's disease. Refer to the treatment for these specific diseases.
- ❐ For bacterial infections use penicillin, penicillin/streptomycin or amoxycillin. Inject twice daily.
- ❐ Move the affected animal to a clean warm well bedded pen.
- ❐ Provide easy access to water or dribble into the mouth three times daily by hose pipe.

Metritis (Endometritis) - Inflammation of the Womb

(Chapter 8 pp252)

Metritis is inflammation of the womb caused by bacterial infection. It is fairly common in the immediate post-farrowing period.

After farrowing the womb contracts and squeezes mucus, white fluid and afterbirth out through the vagina. This discharge can continue for up to 4 days and is normal. If the sow is eating well, has a normal temperature and no mastitis ignore it. However abnormal discharges can also indicate the presence of infection requiring treatment.

Symptoms

Lactating Sows only

- ☞ Temperature.
- ☞ Sow is off her food.
- ☞ Signs of mastitis.

Piglets

- ☞ Starvation - no milk.

- ☞ Bright red mucous membranes around the eyes.
- ☞ Discharge from vulva - white or brown colour.

Causes / Contributing factors

- ◆ Prolonged farrowings.
- ◆ Manual assistance during farrowing.
- ◆ In association with mastitis.
- ◆ Refuses to suckle.

Diagnosis

This is based on the clinical signs.

Treatment

- ❒ Give twice daily injections of antibiotics together with 0.5ml of oxytocin each time.
- ❒ Treatment should be given for 2 to 3 days.
- ❒ If the sow has been assisted at farrowing then an injection of long-acting penicillin is advised at the time to prevent infection.
- ❒ Antibiotics that can be used include OTC, penicillin/streptomycin, amoxycillin, ampicillin, framycetin, trimethoprim/sulpha.

Middle Ear Infections

(Chapter 9 pp319)

This disease occurs occasionally in the sucking pig from 7 to 10 days of age. The middle part of the ear is responsible for balance. The common organisms involved include; *Haemophilus parasuis*, streptococci, and staphylococci. It is more common in the weaned pig and sow.

Symptoms

<u>All Pigs</u>

- ☞ Infection causes the pig to hold its head on the affected side and to lose its balance.
- ☞ May progress to meningitis.
- ☞ Head shaking.

Causes / Contributing factors

- ◆ Sequel to joint infections or septicaemia in piglets.
- ◆ PRRS infection in piglets.
- ◆ Mange/trauma to the ear.

Diagnosis

Early identification of the condition is essential to allow prompt treatment.

Treatment

❒ This should be carried out using daily injections of penicillin/streptomycin, OTC or amoxycillin. It is more common in the weaned pig.

MORTALITY - PIGLETS

(Chapter 8 pp228)

Causes

- This is mainly due to management failures in the first 48 hours after farrowing.

Contributing Factors

- Lack of colostrum / milk.
- Poor teat access.
- Draughts low temperatures.
- Wet pens.
- Scour.
- Poor management.
- Septicaemia.
- Joint infections.

MORTALITY - SOWS

(Chapter 7 pp215)

Sow mortality can be a cause of major economic loss. In approaching this problem first categorise the causes but differentiate between those animals culled on welfare or other grounds and those that actually died.

The range over all herds is 3% - 15%. Levels of 7-9% are not uncommon, at least two thirds of which occur in the dry period. Target levels should be 3% - 6%. of which <2% may be culled on welfare or other grounds.

Causes

- Abscesses.

- Chronic disease.
- Clostridial infections.
- Cystitis / pyelonephritis.
- Dead piglets.
- Electrocution.
- Erysipelas.
- Fighting.
- Fractures.
- Gastric ulcers.
- Heart failure.
- Injury.
- Internal abscesses.
- Internal haemorrhage.
- Lameness.
- Metritis. Womb infection.
- Paralysis.
- Peritonitis.
- Poor body condition.
- Prolapsed rectum.
- Prolapsed uterus.
- Prolapsed vagina.
- Torsion of the stomach or intestines.
- Vulva biting.

Contributing factors

- Age profile of the herd.
- Culling policy.
- Sows sold as culls and not recorded as deaths.
- Breed.
- The stress gene may play a part.
- Variation in body condition.
- Availability of water and the incidence of cystitis/pyelonephritis.
- Sows culled for leg weakness (OCD).
- Parts of the management system that predispose to injury. e.g. mixing.
- Suitability and management of the environment.

- Quality of the feed.
- Feeding system. This may predispose to ruptured or twisted intestines.

Muscle Tearing

This is a common condition in sows in which the muscle fibres are torn away from their attachment to the bones of the inner surfaces of the elbow and knee joints and the pelvis.

Symptoms

Sows

- ☞ Painful inflammation of bone and periosteum.
- ☞ Affected sows often adopt a dog sitting position.
- ☞ Sows cannot stand.

Piglets

- ☞ Piglet can not stand - legs spread laterally.

Causes / Contributing factors

- Torn muscles arise as a sequel to OCD.
- Trauma.
- Fighting.
- Slippery floors.
- Weak bones.
- Splay leg in piglets.

Diagnosis

This is by clinical signs.

Treatment

- ❐ Affected sows should be moved to a solid floor area with deep bedding or to a sheltered grass paddock.

Mycoplasma Arthritis (*Mycoplasma Hyosynoviae* Infection)

(Chapter 9 pp321)

Most herds are infected although not all infected herds show clinical signs. *Mycoplasma hyosynoviae* lives in the upper respiratory tract without causing clinical signs and is spread by droplet infection. It invades the joints and tendon sheaths of susceptible animals and causes lameness and swelling.

Older sows develop a strong immunity which they pass to their offspring in the colostrum.

Infection takes place sometime after this colostral immunity has worn off, usually between 12 and 30 weeks of age but sometimes gilts do not become infected until introduced to a new herd or in early pregnancy.

It is common in purchased gilts which have been reared in isolated grow-outs, but uncommon in mature sows.

Symptoms

Sows/Gilts

- ☞ Clinical signs in the gilt are sudden in onset.
- ☞ Starting with a reluctance to rise.
- ☞ Lameness.
- ☞ Swellings over hock joints visible.
- ☞ Affected pigs are in pain and only stand for short periods.
- ☞ The temperature may be normal or slightly elevated.

Piglets

- ☞ None.
- ☞ Disease rare.
- ☞ Protected by maternal antibody.

Causes / Contributing factors

- The quality of housing - in particular low temperatures and draughts which act as trigger factors.
- Mixing and fighting.
- Respiratory spread.
- High stocking density.
- Sudden reduction in energy intake producing stress.

Diagnosis

This is based on clinical signs and the response to therapy. Joint fluid can be aspirated and examined for antibodies and the organism can be isolated.

Serology is not much help because sub-clinical infection is common and so healthy animals often have antibody titres. Rising titres in blood samples taken two weeks apart aid diagnosis.

Post-mortem examination may be necessary to reach a definitive diagnosis.

It must be differentiated from muscle damage, leg weakness,

trauma, erysipelas, and *Haemophilus parasuis* arthritis.

Treatment

- ❐ Give lincomycin or tiamulin injections daily for 4 days early in the disease. If the lameness is due to *Mycoplasma hyosynoviae* there should be a good response within 24 to 36 hours.
- ❐ Give in feed medication strategically commencing 7 days before the expected disease outbreak and continue for 14 days using 220g/tonne of lincomycin or 500-800g/tonne of OTC.
- ❐ An alternate strategy is to medicate the ration at half these levels and feed for 5-7 weeks.

Navel Bleeding / Pale Pig Syndrome

(Chapter 8 pp272)

At birth or within a few hours the piglet becomes extremely pale and in many cases dies.

Symptoms

Sows

- ☞ Blood may be seen from the vulva.

Piglets

- ☞ Pale pigs.
- ☞ Blood on the floor of the pen arising from the navel.
- ☞ Pigs found dead.

Causes / Contributing factors

The condition arises in one of three ways:

1. The piglet's blood may be pooled into the placenta during farrowing. If the cord is broken at birth, the piglet will be pale and anaemic. Affected piglets are more likely from old sows and in large litters.
2. Pigs are sometimes born with a haemorrhage or a haematoma in the cord itself. The cause of this is unknown but in some cases it is related to premature cord cutting and removal of the piglet from behind the sow at farrowing.
3. Continual bleeding from the navel during the first 3 to 4 hours after birth.

Other factors that predispose:

- Navel bleeding is associated with the use of wood shavings as bedding.

- Warfarin poisoning can be responsible for haemorrhage.
- Mycotoxins from contaminated feed have been implicated
- A riboflavin deficiency has been implicated.
- In some herds there appears to be an association with the use of prostaglandin to synchronise farrowings.
- Do not allow excessive trauma to the cord within 3 hours of birth. This may occur if too many piglets are fastened in the creep area.

Diagnosis

This is by clinical signs.

Treatment

❒ Early recognition of bleeding navel is essential. The cord should be clamped approximately 13mm from the skin using an umbilical clip. Nylon or plastic ties used to bind together electrical wires can also be used.

❒ As an alternative and in an acute emergency the navel can be tied with thin string but it shrinks and the bleeding often continues. The cord should be bent back on itself and re-tied in the shape of a "U".

Oedema of the Udder and Failure of Milk Let Down

(Chapter 8 pp236)

This is a failure of milk let down associated with excess fluid (oedema) in the mammary tissues of all the glands and also between the hind legs and in the vulva. The oedema may lead to mastitis. The pressure in the glands reduces the colostrum so the piglets are not well protected. Subsequent milk flow may be poor and the rear glands may dry off. Piglets receive low colostrum intake and a poor milk supply and waste away. They may scour.

Symptoms

<u>Piglets</u>

☞ Lack of milk.

☞ Scour.

- ☞ Starvation.
- ☞ Increased mortality.

Pre and Post farrowing sows

- ☞ The sow is uncomfortable but does not appear to be in pain.
- ☞ She is otherwise clinically normal.
- ☞ Palpitation of the udder shows fluid either just beneath the skin or deep in the gland and often extending between the legs towards the vulva.

Causes / Contributing factors

- Oedema can be associated with high feed intake, particularly high energy levels.
- A change from straw yards into farrowing houses is associated with a marked reduction in fibre intake.
- Constipation can be a predisposing factor.
- Low water intake 2 to 3 days before farrowing can also predispose.

Diagnosis

This is based on the clinical appearance and palpitation.

Treatment

- ❒ Treat the sow with small doses of oxytocin (0.5 to 1 ml) every 4 to 6 hours on four occasions.
- ❒ Supplement the piglets with artificial milk and make water available in dishes.
- ❒ Give a preventative injection of long-acting penicillin, amoxycillin or OTC if you suspect there are any signs of mastitis.

Osteomalacia (OM)

(Chapter 8 pp251)

This bone condition is due to inadequate levels of calcium phosphorus and or vitamin D. Sows may not be able to absorb sufficient. The density of the bones becomes less and they are prone to fractures particularly mid shaft.

Symptoms

Sows

- ☞ Seen in the first litter gilt.
- ☞ Dog sitting position.

Piglets

- ☞ N/A

- ☞ Stiffness
- ☞ Sudden acute lameness during lactation or immediately post weaning.

Causes / Contributing factors

- ◆ Inadequate diet.
- ◆ Heavy milk production.
- ◆ Low feed intake in lactation.
- ◆ Breed of animal.

Diagnosis

This is by the clinical signs. Can be confused with OCD and fractures.

Treatment

- ❒ Give vitamin D injection to gilts at farrowing.
- ❒ Add calcium phosphorus supplement to the diet daily during lactation.
- ❒ Destroy affected sows with fractures.

Parasites

(Chapter 11 pp369)

In the sow the important worms are the large white worms ascarids (*Ascaris suum*), red stomach worms (*Hyostrongylus rubidus*) and whip worms (*Trichuris suis*). The sow becomes the source of potential infection to piglets. The threadworm (*Strongyloides ransomi*) is important in the piglet. The life cycles of all are direct from eggs in faeces to adult in the intestine.

Symptoms

Sows

- ☞ Coughing.
- ☞ Loss of body condition.
- ☞ Vomiting.
- ☞ Blood in faeces.
- ☞ Anaemia.
- ☞ Diarrhoea.

Piglets (Thread Worm)

- ☞ Coughing.
- ☞ Stiffness.
- ☞ Pain.
- ☞ Vomiting.
- ☞ Bloody diarrhoea.
- ☞ Some mortality.

Causes / Contributing factors

- ◆ Management systems that allow regular access to faeces.

- Faeces allowed to accumulate for more than 3 - 4 days (allows eggs to become infective).
- Moist wet areas encourage survival of eggs.
- No all-in, all-out management.
- Permanently populated yards or paddocks outdoors.
- Failure to monitor faeces for egg output.
- Failure to carry out routine treatments when indicated.

Diagnosis

This is based on symptoms and identification of the parasites. Examinations of faeces samples.

Treatment

❒ Use broad spectrum anthelmintics, ideally in feed or by injection.

❒ Compounds available include doramectin, ivermectin, fenbendazole, flubendazole, oxfendazole, oxibendazole and thiophanate

Peritonitis

(Chapter 7 pp217)

Peritonitis is inflammation of the peritoneum, the shiny membrane that covers all the internal surfaces in the abdomen. The onset may be sudden or gradual. A common time is 7-10 days after damage by the boar at mating per vagina. It may arise due to a septicaemia.

Symptoms

Sows / Growers

☞ Abdominal pain.

☞ Appetite normal or depressed.

☞ The sow is reluctant to move.

☞ Loses weight.

☞ Has a tucked up appearance.

☞ A discharge from the vulva may be apparent at mating.

☞ The temperature may be normal or elevated.

Piglets

☞ Swollen abdomen.

☞ Wasting.

☞ Death.

Causes / Contributing factors

- Ruptured gastric ulcer.
- Perforated bowel.
- Penetration of the abdomen via mating.

- External trauma to the abdomen and ruptured bowel or liver.
- Conditions such as actinobacillus pleuropneumonia, migrating ascarid worms, miscellaneous generalised infections may also result in peritonitis.

Diagnosis

This is based on the clinical signs and history. A post-mortem examination may be required to confirm it.

Treatment

❒ Treatment is by broad spectrum antibiotics for 5 to 7 days. Inject with either OTC, penicillin, streptomycin or amoxycillin.

❒ The response is usually poor.

Pneumonia (Chronic Respiratory Disease)

(Chapter 7 pp217)

Pneumonia is normally uncommon in mature acclimatised animals (unless exposed to a new organism) but occasionally it occurs in gilts. Mortality in naive animals can be as high as 10 to 15% (no immunity) if prompt treatment is not undertaken.

The onset of swine influenza is usually sudden. The onset of enzootic pneumonia in a naive herd may be insidious although it may later develop rapidly affecting many sows severely. There is likely to be severe pneumonia and some mortality if the disease is not controlled in herds infected for the first time.

Symptoms

Sows

☞ Widespread coughing.

☞ Some sows obviously very ill.

☞ Respiratory rate is elevated, some showing acute respiratory distress.

Piglets

☞ Coughing.

☞ Heavy breathing.

☞ Loss of condition.

☞ Dehydration.

Causes / Contributing factors

- If pathogens such as influenza, PRRS virus, *Mycoplasma hyopneumoniae* or a virulent strain of *Actinobacillus pleuropneumoniae* enter a susceptible herd for the first time dramatic, outbreaks may occur in sows.

- Poor environments.
- Incorrect ventilation and humidity.
- High stocking densities.

Diagnosis

This is based on the clinical signs and post-mortem examinations. Laboratory tests involving serology and microbiology are often necessary to identify the precise causes.

Treatment

- ❒ Broad spectrum antibiotics such as OTC, penicillin streptomycin or amoxycillin are indicated.
- ❒ Inject individual cases daily for 3 to 4 days.
- ❒ For influenza outbreaks with secondary bacteria:
  - Combine CTC or OTC in the water at the onset together with in-feed medication at a level of 600g/tonne.
  - Antibiotic cover is required for at least 14 to 21 days.
- ❒ For enzootic pneumonia, drugs effective against mycoplasma are indicated
  - Lincomycin - In feed, water, or by injection.
  - Spectinomycin - By injection.
  - Tiamulin - In feed, water, or by injection.
  - Tylosin - In feed, water, or by injection.
  - Chlortetracycline - In feed, or water.
  - Oxytetracycline - In feed, water, or by injection.
- ❒ It is important in the early stages of a breakdown until an immunity has developed, to control the numbers of organisms shed into the air. This can be achieved by using 600-800g/tonne of OTC or CTC in feed for two weeks reducing this to 200 to 300g over the next 3 to 4 weeks.
- ❒ For actinobacillus pleuropneumonia early treatment of individuals with OTC, penicillin/streptomycin, ceftiofur or sulphonamides is necessary together with preventative medication in-feed or water.

Porcine Cytomegalovirus Infection (PCMV)

(Chapter 6 pp170)

This is a herpes virus found in the tissues throughout the body including the nose of newborn piglets where it causes inflammation (rhinitis). PCMV is present throughout the world and exists in most if not all pig populations but most infections are sub-clinical and clinical disease is rare. Serology carried out in the UK, for example, indicates that over 90% of herds have been exposed to infection.

The rhinitis produced by this virus is uncommon and occurs mainly in newborn pigs and has no relationship to atrophic rhinitis caused by the toxin-producing bacteria *Pasteurella multocidia*. In most herds therefore the infection is insignificant and apart from sometimes causing a mild sneeze has no major effect on the health of the pig.

Symptoms

Piglets / Weaners only

- ☞ Rhinitis in newborn piglets can be severe enough to cause haemorrhage from the nose.
- ☞ In herds in which PCMV is endemic there are no symptoms other than mild sneezing in sucking and weaned piglets.

Sows

- ☞ Clinical signs are only seen if PCMV infects a sow for the first time when she is late in pregnancy.
- ☞ Foetal deaths.
- ☞ Mummified foetuses.
- ☞ Stillbirths.
- ☞ Weak piglets.
- ☞ A slight fever .
- ☞ Inappetence.
- ☞ Nasal haemorrhage.

Causes / Contributing factors

- The virus is shed in discharges from the nose and eyes, urine and farrowing fluids.

- It is also transmitted via the boar through semen and crosses the placenta to infect piglets before birth.
- Poor environmental conditions.
- Fluctuating temperatures may predispose.
- Dust.
- Continually populated houses.

Diagnosis

This can be confirmed by serological tests, fluorescent antibody tests and demonstration of inclusion bodies in tissue sections.

The disease might be confused with atrophic rhinitis or bordetella infection of the nose, however the effects are very short lived and there is no progressive atrophy or distortion of the nose.

PCMV rhinitis only occurs in newborn piglets and there is a tendency to assume that sneezing in piglets must be associated with atrophic rhinitis. Rhinitis means inflammation of the delicate tissues in the nose and is caused by dust, gases, bacteria or viruses, in fact any irritant. If toxin producing pasteurella are present the inflammation persists with damage and progressive destruction of the tissues (atrophy). This is a serious disease. It can be differentiated from PCMV by swabbing the noses of sneezing piglets and testing for the presence or absence of the pasteurella. It is important to carry this out because if the tests are negative you have no worries (or expensive treatments).

Treatment

- ❒ None is required.
- ❒ If sneezing and poor growth occur post-weaning, the creep can be medicated with antibiotics such as CTC, OTC, trimethoprim/sulpha or tylosin for 14 days.

Porcine Enteropathy (PE)

(Chapter 9 pp324)

PE takes 4 forms. All are uncommon in the mature female but outbreaks of one of the forms, bloody gut or porcine haemorrhagic enteropathy (PHE), is common in maiden and pregnant gilts.

Symptoms

Sows

- ☞ Gilts with PHE have pale skins.
- ☞ Appear weak.
- ☞ Bloody or black tarry diarrhoea.
- ☞ May suddenly die.

Piglets

- ☞ N/A

Causes / Contributing factors

These are not fully understood.

- ◆ The use of continually populated pens.
- ◆ Lack of all-in, all-out production.
- ◆ Naive animal.
- ◆ Change of environment.
- ◆ Changes in feed.

Diagnosis

Laboratory examinations of small intestine. A bloody swollen intestine (the terminal part) is indicative.

Treatment

- ❐ Feed medication with tetracyclines or tylosin is a common preventive measure.

Porcine Epidemic Diarrhoea (PED)

(Chapter 12 pp410)

Porcine epidemic diarrhoea is caused by a coronavirus somewhat similar to that which causes TGE. This virus is widespread in Europe. The virus damages the villi in the gut thus reducing the absorptive surface, with loss of fluid and dehydration. After introduction of the virus into a susceptible breeding herd, a strong immunity develops over two to three weeks. The colostral immunity then protects the piglets. The virus usually disappears spontaneously from breeding herds particularly small ones (< 300 sows).

Acute outbreaks of diarrhoea occur when the virus is first introduced into a susceptible population. In such cases up to 100% of sows may be affected, showing a mild to very watery diarrhoea. Two clinical pictures are recognised: PED Type I only affects growing pigs whereas PED Type II affects all ages including sucking pigs and mature sows. The incubation period is approximately 2 days and diarrhoea lasts for 7 to 14 days. In sucking pigs the disease can be mild or severe with mortalities up to 40%.

In large breeding herds, particularly if kept extensively, not all the females may become infected first time round and there may be recrudescence. This only occurs in piglets suckling from sows with no maternal antibodies and is therefore sporadic.

Symptoms

Sows

- This can vary from very mild "cow pat" faeces through to a watery diarrhoea.
- Loose faeces.

Piglets

- Diarrhoea.
- Dehydration.

Causes / Contributing factors

- The immunological status of the herd i.e. no immunity.

Diagnosis

If acute diarrhoea is occurring in weaned and older animals with no symptoms in sucking piglets it suggests PED Type I. PED type II may be suspected on the clinical signs if mild, but it cannot be differentiated from TGE. Blood tests can be carried out to look for rising antibody titres. An ELISA test and fluorescent antibody test (FAT) are used for examining diarrhoea samples or intestinal wall and contents.

Treatment

- Because this is a virus infection there is no specific treatment.
- If the virus enters the herd for the first time it is important to ensure that all the adult animals become infected at an early stage to allow an early immunity to develop. This can be achieved by exposing sows to the diarrhoea via the drinking water. Mix scour or contaminated material into a bucket of water and use this as the source.

Porcine Parvovirus Infection (PPV)

(Chapter 6 pp170)

This is the most common and important cause of infectious infertility. Porcine parvovirus is a fairly tough virus that multiplies normally in the intestine of the pig without causing clinical signs. It is world-wide in its distribution. If you test for it in your pig herd it is almost certain it will be present unless your herd is less than 100 sows when it might have died out. It is therefore an infection you have to live with and manage. Whereas most viruses do not survive outside the host for any great period of time PPV is unusual in that it can persist outside the pig for many months and it is resistant to most disinfectants. This perhaps explains why it is so widespread and so difficult to remove from the pig environment.

Symptoms

Piglets

- None normally.
- Occasional low visible ones are seen.
- Increase in stillbirths associated with mummified piglets.

Sows

- Small litters associated with embryo loss before 35 days.
- Mummified pigs of varying size, (30-160mm).
- Increased numbers of stillbirths.
- These are associated with the delay in the farrowing mechanism which occurs because of the presence of the mummified piglet.
- Abortions associated with PPV infection are uncommon.
- There may be an increase in low birth weight piglets but neonatal deaths are not affected.
- The acute disease episode often lasts for up to 8 weeks then wanes for 4-6 weeks, followed by smaller bouts of mummified pigs for a further 4-6 weeks.
- The virus can take up to 4 months to infect all sows in a susceptible previously uninfected herd.
- Sporadic disease is seen in individual females which are infected for the first time. It is usually confined to gilts.
- No other signs of ill health in the breeding female or in individual affected animals.

Immunity

PPV infection results in high antibody levels in the serum which persist for long periods. You should appreciate that such levels do not necessarily mean that there is or has been a reproductive problem or a higher level of protection. For example, a titre of 1:2 will be equally as protective as a titre of 1:80,000. Blood sampling all the sows in a herd on one occasion only indicates the percentage of animals that have been exposed to parvovirus at some previous period which gives you an idea of the overall breeding herd immunity or susceptibility. Once an animal has been exposed to PPV it remains immune for the rest of its life.

Key points to parvovirus infection

- The virus is widespread throughout all pig populations but it may disappear in small herds (<100 sows).
- Infection is endemic (present all the time) in most pig units.
- Once a pig is exposed there is a lifelong immunity.
- Reproductive problems may appear every 3-4 years in a herd if vaccination is not carried out.
- Parvovirus infection in a susceptible female can cause death of the embryo with absorption or death of the foetus with mummification.
- The major signs are therefore small litter sizes, mummified pigs of different sizes, and increases in pseudo-pregnancies and not-in-pigs.
- Abortion due to PPV is uncommon.
- Maternal immunity may persist up to 7 months of age but only in a few gilts. (This interferes with vaccine response).
- Up to 50% of gilts may be sero-negative at point of mating.

Causes / Contributing factors

- ◆ In small herds the virus may die out and sows become susceptible.
- ◆ In large herds,pockets of naive breeding females, particularly gilts, can maintain the disease.

Diagnosis

In the absence of any other signs of illness in the breeding females, PPV disease can be suspected by increases in variable sized mummified pigs and small litter sizes.

The important features are disease and death in the embryo and foetus from approximately 15-70 days of pregnancy. The mummified pigs can be examined by fluorescent antibody test in the laboratory to confirm the infection. Serology will not help because many sows are positive and normal.

Treatment

- There is no treatment.
- Vaccination is very effective in preventing disease.

Eradication

Parvovirus can be eradicated from a herd (e.g. sometimes by SEW) but it is not advisable to attempt it.

Porcine Reproductive and Respiratory Syndrome (PRRS)

(Chapter 6 pp173)

The virus of PRRS has a particular affinity for the macrophages particularly those found in the lung. Macrophages are part of the body defences. They ingest and remove invading bacteria and viruses but not in the case of the PRRS virus. Instead, the virus multiplies inside them producing more virus and kills the macrophages. Once it has entered a herd it tends to remain present and active indefinitely.

It may take up to a year for all breeding stock, particularly in large herds, to become infected for the first time and although the virus appears to spread rapidly in a herd it may be some 4 -5 months before at least 90% of the sows have become sero-positive. Some sows remain naive. Furthermore, it is not uncommon for sow herds 1-2 years after infection to contain less than 20% of serological positive animals. This does not however necessarily mean they are not still immune nor does it mean that they have stopped passing on immunity to their offspring. Adult animals shed virus for much shorter periods of time (14 days) compared to growing pigs which can excrete for 1-2 months.

The clinical picture can vary tremendously from one herd to another. As a guide, for every three herds that are exposed to PRRS for the first time one will show no recognisable disease, the second would show mild disease and the third moderate to severe disease.

The reasons for this are not clearly understood. However the higher the health status of the herd, the less severe are the disease effects. It may be that the virus is mutating as it multiplies, throwing up some strains that are highly virulent and some that are not.

Symptoms

Acute disease

- ☞ When the virus first enters the breeding herd disease is seen in dry sows, lactating sows and sucking piglets.

Clinical signs in dry sows during the first month of infection

- ☞ Short periods of inappetence spreading over 7-14 days, 10-15% of sows at any one time.
- ☞ The body temperature may be elevated to 39-40°C (103-105°F).
- ☞ Abortions, often late term, may occur at a 1-6% level. These are often the first signs to be noted.
- ☞ Transient discoloration (blueing) of the ears may be seen (2% level. Blue ear disease).
- ☞ Some sows farrow slightly early. 10-15% over the first 4 weeks.
- ☞ Increased returns occur 21-35 days post-service.
- ☞ Prolonged anoestrus and delayed returns to heat post-weaning.
- ☞ Coughing and respiratory signs.

Clinical signs in farrowing sows in the first month of infection

- ☞ Inappetence over the farrowing period.
- ☞ A reluctance to drink.
- ☞ Agalactia and mastitis - significant symptoms.
- ☞ Farrowings are often 2-3 days early.
- ☞ Discoloration of the skin and pressure sores associated with small vesicles.
- ☞ Lethargy.
- ☞ Respiratory signs.
- ☞ Mummified piglets. 10-15% may die in the last 3-4 weeks of pregnancy.
- ☞ Stillbirth levels increase up to 30%.
- ☞ Very weak piglets at birth.
- ☞ The initial phase of inappetence and fever will often take 3-6 weeks to move through.

- ☞ Cyanosis or blueing of the ears is a variable finding and less than 5% of sows show it. It is transient and may last for only a few hours.
- ☞ Coughing occurs in some sows and a few individual cases of clinical pneumonia may occur.
- ☞ This acute phase lasts in the herd for up to 6 weeks, and is characterised by early farrowings, increases in stillbirths, weak pigs and an increase in the numbers of large mummified pigs that have died in the last three weeks of pregnancy. In some herds, these may reach up to 30% of the total pigs born. Piglet mortality peaks at 70% in weeks 3 or 4 after the onset of symptoms and only returns to pre-infected levels after 8-12 weeks. The reproductive problems may persist for 4-8 months before returning to normal, however in some herds it may actually improve on the pre-PRRS performance.
- ☞ Longer term effects of PRRS on reproductive efficiency are difficult to assess, particularly in herds of low health status. In some there are increases in repeat matings, vulval discharges and abortions, all of which may be blamed on PRRS.
- ☞ The effects of PRRS on reproduction efficiency in herds in which the infection has become enzootic have been observed in the field for up to 12 months after disease has apparently settled.

  These are as follows:
  - A 10-15% reduction in farrowing rate (90% of herds return to normality).
  - Reduced numbers born alive.
  - Increased stillbirths.
  - Poor reproduction in gilts.
  - Early farrowings.
  - Increased levels of abortion (2-3%).
  - Inappetence in sows at farrowing.

Piglets

- ☞ More diarrhoea.
- ☞ Less viable piglets.
- ☞ Increase in respiratory infections such as glässers disease.

Signs in boars

- ☞ Inappetence.
- ☞ Increased body temperature.
- ☞ Lethargy.
- ☞ Loss of libido.
- ☞ Lowered fertility.
- ☞ Poor litter sizes.
- ☞ Lowered sperm output.

Causes / Contributing factors

The following are common methods of spread.

- Movement of carrier pigs.
- Airborne transmission up to 3km (2 miles).
- Mechanical means via faeces, dust, droplets and contaminated equipment, lorries etc.
- Contaminated boots and clothing.
- Vehicles especially in cold weather.
- Artificial insemination but only if the boar is viraemic. This period is probably only 3-4 days.
- The mallard duck and probably other species of bird.
- PRRS infects all types of herd including high or ordinary health status and both indoor and outdoor units, irrespective of size.

Diagnosis

If the herd has not been exposed to PRRS then blood sampling and testing a minimum of 12 adult animals (preferably those that have been off their food at least three weeks) provides a reliable means of diagnosis.

Treatment

There is no treatment as yet available in animals against virus infections. With PRRS however, it is essential during the acute phase to prevent the multiplication of bacteria that normally would have been destroyed by macrophages. Antibiotic treatment should be given for 3-4 weeks to all sows and boars immediately the disease is diagnosed or suspected. If necessary commence with water soluble antibiotics followed by in-feed medication. Prompt treatment usually reduces abortions, stillbirths, mummified pigs and early farrowings caused by secondary bacteria.

Treatment of sows during acute disease

- ❒ Medicate the sow's feed immediately with 500g/tonne of tetracycline either CTC or OTC for at least 4 weeks.
- ❒ If sows are inappetent, medicate the water with OTC or CTC at the onset.
- ❒ Apply the medication to both gilts and boars.
- ❒ Inject individual sows with long-acting OTC or penicillin during periods of inappetence or as advised by your veterinarian.
- ❒ Give long-acting preparations of antibiotics to sows at farrowing. Oxytetracycline or semi-synthetic penicillins are drugs of choice.
- ❒ Alternatively top dress the sows food daily with in-feed antibiotics premixes. Use OTC, CTC or TMS. (Give 15-20g of a 10% premix per day).

Management control includes good nursing and the provision of improved environments for the pigs during the acute periods.

A farm can be depopulated cleaned, disinfected and repopulated with PRRS negative stock. Depopulation is very expensive and before considering this investigate how the herd became infected in the first place and assess the chances off it being re infected again. Repopulation should not be attempted in winter because as the temperature drops, the survival of the virus increases, e.g. 24 hours at 37ºC (99ºF), 6 days at 20ºC (68ºF), one month at 4ºC (39ºF). The virus is stable when frozen for long periods of time.

Porcine Respiratory Corona Virus Infection (PRCV)

(Chapter 9 pp326 and Chapter 12 pp411))

PRCV first appeared in pigs in Europe some ten years or more ago. It is related to but distinct from TGE virus, which is another corona virus. It is thought to spread between farms on wind and so it is extremely difficult to keep herds free from it. Infection often takes place in the sucking pig at 2 to 3 weeks of age but is not of importance. It may have an effect on lung tissue when other respiratory pathogens are present in chronic respiratory disease complexes.

Symptoms

Sows

☞ Usually no symptoms.
☞ In the presence of other respiratory agents coughing may be associated.

Piglets

☞ A transient cough but no other signs.

Causes / Contributing factors

- Field observations indicate the virus is spread for long distances on the wind.

Diagnosis

PRCV cross reacts with TGE in standard serological tests and therefore can confuse the diagnosis. A differential test is available which distinguishes between the two but some recent results have proved positive indicating a possible new virus or altered strain of TGE.

Treatment

❒ None necessary.

Porcine Spongiform Encephalopathy (PSE)

No naturally occurring cases of this have been identified in the pig. It has been produced experimentally by direct inoculation of infected bovine brain tissue into the brain. Feeding infected brain tissue however has not resulted in disease. The feeding of meat and bone meal to pigs is now banned in the UK but during its use no cases have been identified.

Porcine Stress Syndrome (PSS)

(Chapter 7 pp218)

This term covers a group of conditions associated with a recessive gene. The group includes acute stress and sudden death (malignant hyperthermia), pale soft exudative muscle (PSE), dark firm dry meat, and back muscle necrosis. Heavy muscled pigs are more likely to carry the gene than leaner pigs. The gene is called the halothane gene because of the adverse effect halothane anaesthetic has on pigs carrying it. Each pig is homozygous (i.e. possessing a pair of halothane genes), or heterozygous (i..e. possessing one normal gene and one halothane gene) or two normal genes. Homozygous pigs or their meat may show any of the four conditions.

Homozygous (but not heterozygous) pigs can be identified by their response to the anaesthetic with halothane. Recent developments have produced a gene probe that identifies both the homozygous and heterozygous carriers using only a drop of blood or a single hair. Back muscle necrosis is a more localised form of PSS.

When the homozygous state is present and following a period of muscle activity, there is a change in muscle metabolism from aerobic to anaerobic and biochemical abnormalities develop. The body tissues become acid with a marked rise in temperature 42°C (107°F).

Symptoms

Sows

The onset is sudden with:

- ☞ Marked muscle tremors.
- ☞ Twitching of the face.
- ☞ Rapid respiration.
- ☞ The skin becomes red and blotched.
- ☞ Death usually occurs within 15-20 minutes.
- ☞ Rigor mortis (stiffening of the muscles after death) within 5 minutes is a striking feature.
- ☞ Rise in temperature.

Piglets

- ☞ Rarely seen.
- ☞ If so as in sows.

Causes / Contributing factors

- Disease is precipitated by sudden muscle activity.
- The carrier pig is genetically susceptible.

Diagnosis

This is based on the sudden onset, clinical signs, breed susceptibility and the known presence or absence of the gene in the pig.

In many cases the pig is just found dead and a post-mortem examination is necessary to eliminate other diseases. These include other causes of sudden death, twisted bowel, internal haemorrhage, mulberry heart disease, cystitis/pyelonephritis and hypocalcaemia.

Treatment

Treatment is usually ineffective but the following are worth trying:

❒ Spray the pig with cold water..

❒ Inject 50-100ml of calcium gluconate intramuscularly injections at two sites. Seek veterinary advice.

❒ Sedate the pig with stresnil.

❒ Do not move or cause undue muscle activity.

❒ Give an injection of vitamin E 2iu/kg.

Prepucial Ulceration

(Chapter 10 pp362)

This is occasionally seen in outdoor boars and may become a problem in groups of boars. It appears to spread slowly.

Symptoms

Boars

☞ The skin around the prepucial opening is red and inflamed and is clearly evident when the boar is still.

Causes / Contributing factors

The cause is unknown but it may be initiated by:

- Trauma.
- Viral or bacterial infections.
- Contact dermatitis.

Diagnosis

This is by the clinical signs.

Treatment

❒ Because the cause is unknown and the possibility that the condition may spread between boars and sows, it is advisable to cull affected animals immediately.

❒ Alternatively isolate animals, treat with antibiotics by injections and spray the prepuce with iodine cow teat dip.

❒ Healing takes place over 4 - 6 weeks after which infection probably has disappeared.

Prolapse of the Bladder

(Chapter 8 pp253)

This is an uncommon condition. The bladder turns inside out and protrudes from the lips of the vulva.

Symptoms

Piglets

☞ N/A

Sows

☞ The inside of the bladder appears as a large red mass about the size of an orange.

☞ It can be confused with an early prolapse of the uterus but examination will show that is like a small balloon.

Causes / Contributing factors

◆ It arises when there is a large urethral opening at the floor of the vagina and complete loss of muscle tone in the sphincter.

Diagnosis

Veterinary advice is suggested if in doubt. It can be confused with vaginal prolapse and vaginal polyps.

Treatment

❒ The everted bladder can usually be returned to its former position using obstetrical fluid. The tissues are gently pushed back into the vagina and the bladder returned. This is probably a task for your veterinarian.

❒ Give antibiotic cover by injections for 3 days such as trimethoprim/sulpha.

Prolapse of the Rectum

(Chapter 9 pp327)

This is not uncommon in sows.

Symptoms

Piglets

☞ Rare.

☞ As for sows.

Sows

☞ At the onset, the red coloured mucosa of the rectum protrudes from the anal sphincter.

- May return on its own or remain to the exterior, become swollen and filled with fluid.
- It is prone to damage, haemorrhage and cannibalism.
- Pale pigs due to haemorrhage.

Causes / Contributing factors

The exact mechanisms are not understood but the following should be considered as contributory factors.

- Prolapses which occur after oestrus may be related to sex hormone levels.
- Prolapses may occur with constipation e.g. from feeding a low fibre diet.
- Penetration of the rectum at mating may result in prolapse 24-48 hours later.
- Stalls or tethers with an excessive slope of the floor towards the back.
- Sow stalls or farrowing crates with the back retaining gate consisting of parallel bars seem to predispose. If the sow can rest with the tail over the back gait, pressure is placed on the anus. This causes a partial relaxation of the sphincter, poor circulation and swelling. The sow strains and prolapses.
- Prolapsed rectum may occur whenever there is an increase in abdominal pressure, for example a sow laying over the edge of small raised lying area in confinement.
- Abnormal fermentation in the gut and the production of gas in the large bowel may predispose. In such cases the components of the feed and the method of feeding should be investigated.
- Mouldy feeds or straw containing mycotoxins can cause rectal prolapses.
- Shortage of water may predispose.
- Genetic factors do not appear to have a part to play in this condition.

Diagnosis

This is by the clinical signs.

Treatment

- This consists of replacing the prolapse and retaining it with a suture around the rectum. The procedure for carrying this out is described in *Chapter 15 pp 501.*

- ❒ Where outbreaks occur a change in ration or the inclusion of 200g of CTC in feed for a short period will often be sufficient to control the condition. The CTC suppresses those organisms that cause fermentation and gas production in the large bowel.

Prolapse of the Uterus (womb)

(Chapter 15 pp504)

This involves the complete eversion of both horns of the womb which turn completely inside out. It usually takes place within 2-4 hours of the completion of farrowing but sometimes up to 24 hours afterwards. Prolonged straining causes a small part of the tube to be propelled outwards by uterine contractions.

Symptoms

<u>Sows</u>

- ☞ The prolapse occurs over a period of approximately one hour and commences with the appearance of the red congested lining of the womb.
- ☞ This rapidly increases in size until the large everted mass is presented.

Causes / Contributing factors

- ◆ Uterine prolapses are uncommon but usually occur in old sows with large litters or where large piglets have been born.
- ◆ The supporting structures of the uterus become weak or the uterine wall becomes flaccid.

Diagnosis

This is obvious by the appearance.

Treatment

- ❒ Treatment involves replacing the womb inside the sow. This is often impossible or the sow dies from internal haemorrhage.
- ❒ The technique for carrying this out is discussed in *Chapter 15 pp 504.*
- ❒ Under most circumstances the sow should be destroyed on welfare grounds.

Prolapse of the Vagina and Cervix

(Chapter 6 pp220)

Prolapse of the vagina and cervix commonly occurs in the last third of pregnancy including the immediate pre-farrowing period.

Symptoms

Sows

☞ In the early stages the protruding tissues appear between the lips of the vulva and return to their normal position when the sow stands.

☞ With advancing pregnancy the prolapse may remain to the exterior and as soon as this occurs the animal should be removed from it's existing environment and loose-housed.

☞ The tissues become swollen with time.

Causes / Contributing factors

- It occurs usually in older fatter sows that are heavy in pig.
- It is a response to increased abdominal pressure together with a relaxation of the internal structures that support the neck of the womb.
- It is more common in older sows.
- Sows housed on tethers with slippery floors are more prone.
- Stalls or tethers with floors that slopes too steeply to the rear predispose.
- High levels of starchy feed intake, produce excess fermentation and gas and an increase in abdominal pressure.

Diagnosis

This is by clinical signs. It may be confused with eversion of the bladder but may be differentiated by handling the tissues.

Treatment

❒ Remove the sow to loose housing.

❒ If the prolapse remains when the sow is standing replace it and pass a tape suture across the vulva. The procedure for carrying this out is described in *Chapter 15 pp 503*.

❒ If the sow is at point of farrowing, the farrowing crate floor should be raised to slope towards the feeding trough by using raised floor boards. When the sow then stands or lies down the weight of the piglets inside pulls the womb forward to hold the vagina in. Under such circumstances the sow usually farrows normally.

❐ If the vagina remains prolapsed as farrowing approaches, the cervix will not open fully and both the sow and the litter are likely to be lost. In such cases a tape suture should be placed across the lips of the vulva to hold the prolapse in. As the sow reaches the point of farrowing it can be relaxed.

Rabies

This is caused by a virus and considered a rare disease in pigs. It is invariably fatal in all species including the human - hence its importance. Rabies is absent from the UK but present in may other countries throughout the world.

Symptoms

Sows

Onset is sudden with:

- ☞ Nervous twitching of the face muscles.
- ☞ Rapid chewing.
- ☞ Salivation.
- ☞ The muscles may also go into spasm.
- ☞ Posterior paralysis may occur.
- ☞ Death usually takes place within 3 days.

Piglets

- ☞ Rare.
- ☞ As for sows.

Causes / Contributing factors

- ◆ Rabies virus is spread by contact with wild life.

Diagnosis

Consult your veterinarian immediately.

Treatment

❐ There is no treatment.

Rotavirus Infection

(Chapter 7 pp274)

This virus is widespread in pig populations. It is present in most if not all pig herds with virtually a 100% sero-conversion in adult stock. A further epidemiological feature is its persistence outside the pig where it is resistant to environmental changes and many disinfectants. Maternal antibodies persist for 3-6 weeks after which pigs become susceptible to infection but exposure does not necessarily result in disease. It is estimated that only 10-15% of diarrhoeas in pigs are initiated by a primary rotavirus infection. In a mature herd disease appears after piglets are 7 to 10 days of age. It becomes progressively less important with age. However if pathogenic strains of *E. coli* are present severe disease can occur with heavy mortality.

Symptoms

Sows

☞ Transient diarrhoea.

Piglets

☞ Watery profuse diarrhoea in younger animals.
☞ Villus atrophy is a consistent feature with dehydration and mal-absorption.
☞ Diarrhoea usually persists for 3-4 days.
☞ Pigs look hollow in the abdomen.
☞ The eyes are sunken.
☞ The skin around the rectum is wet.

Causes / Contributing factors

- Poor house hygiene.
- Permanently populated houses. Adopt all-in, all-out.
- Movement of pigs.
- Temperature fluctuations.
- Contaminated boots and clothing.

Diagnosis

Whenever there is a diarrhoea problem in pigs over 7 days of age rotavirus identification is required by electron microscopy and ELISA tests. Try the litmus test. Soak scour in litmus paper, *E. coli* infections turn blue, virus infections red.

Treatment

❒ There is no specific treatment.
❒ Provide antibiotic therapy either by injection, by mouth or in the drinking water, to control secondary infections such as *E. coli.*

- ❐ Apralan, amoxycillin, neomycin, framycetin and enrofloxacin could be used.
- ❐ Provide dextrose/glycine electrolytes to counteract dehydration.
- ❐ Provide dry warm and comfortable lying areas.

SALMONELLOSIS

(Chapter 9 pp334)

Salmonella bacteria are widespread in human and animal populations. Some of them can cause disease in pigs.

They multiply mainly in the intestines of young growing pigs but also in some sows. They may be shed in faeces for several weeks or months with no clinical disease. Salmonella in the gut of the pig can contaminate carcasses during the slaughter process and their presence creates potential public health risks from food poisoning.

Salmonella choleraesuis and *Salmonella derby* are host-adapted to the pig and may be carried for long periods by sows, the former sometimes causing clinical disease in sows (fever, depression, septicaemia, pneumonia, meningitis arthritis and diarrhoea) but rarely in people. The serotype most commonly found in pigs, however, is *Salmonella typhimurium* which sometimes is associated with diarrhoea in young pigs but which is also a major cause of food poisoning in people. Some strains have multiple drug resistance. If it is diagnosed in your pigs you should take hygienic precautions not to become infected yourself. Many other so called exotic types may also be detected in pigs without causing disease.

Disease is dose dependent, that is, a relatively large number of organisms are required before clinical signs occur.

Symptoms

Piglets

- ☞ Disease would be uncommon in the piglet and due to passive immunity provided via colostrum.

Sows

- ☞ Clinical signs of *Salmonella choleraesuis* and occasionally *Salmonella typhimurium* infection may include any combination of the following:

- ☞ A high temperature.
- ☞ Depression.
- ☞ Loss of appetite.
- ☞ Congestion of the ears, snout and tail.
- ☞ Pneumonia.
- ☞ Coughing.
- ☞ Nervous signs.
- ☞ A smelly sometimes bloody diarrhoea.
- ☞ Death may occur in the acute phase of the disease.

Causes / Contributing factors

- ◆ Poor hygiene.
- ◆ Overcrowding.
- ◆ Stress by moving and mixing.
- ◆ Permanently populated houses.
- ◆ Contaminated boots and clothing.
- ◆ Mechanical means via faeces and the movement of contaminated equipment.
- ◆ Vermin and flies.
- ◆ Contamination of feed by birds, rats and mice.
- ◆ Contamination of raw feed ingredients and thus the final product.

Diagnosis

This is carried out by culturing the organism either from the faeces, or from the internal organs of dead pigs.

Treatment

- ❒ Treatment is rarely necessary in the sow.
- ❒ Antibiotics could be used in feed to reduce infection levels.

SALT POISONING - (WATER DEPRIVATION)

(Chapter 7 pp221)

Salt poisoning is common in all ages of pig and is related to shortage of water availability. The normal levels of salt in the diet (0.4-0.5%) become toxic in the absence of water.

It should be a daily routine to check that all sources of water are adequate, free flowing and available.

Symptoms

All Pigs

- ☞ The very early stages of disease are preceded by inappetence. Whenever a sow or group of pigs are not eating always check the water supply first. Signs develop within 24 to 48 hours.
- ☞ The first signs are often pigs trying to drink from nipple drinkers unsuccessfully.
- ☞ Nervous signs then develop with fits and animals wandering around apparently blind.
- ☞ Often a pig walks up to a wall, stands and presses its head against it.
- ☞ One sign strongly suggestive of salt poisoning is nose twitching just before a convulsion starts.

Causes / Contributing factors

- Water shortage/deprivation.
- Excess salt in the diet.

Diagnosis

This is based upon the clinical signs and lack of water. Examination of the brain histologically at post-mortem confirms the disease.

Salt poisoning must be differentiated from Aujeszky's disease, swine fever, streptococcal meningitis and middle ear infection but this only affects one individual rather than a group.

Treatment

- ❒ Treatment is not very effective but involves rehydrating the animal. At a practical level this can be achieved by dripping water into the mouth of the pig through a hose pipe or alternatively via a flutter valve into the rectum where it is absorbed. *(Chapter 15 pp 486).*
- ❒ Discuss the possibility of administering sterile water into the abdomen with your veterinarian.
- ❒ Corticosteroids may also help.

Savaging of Piglets (Cannibalism)

(Chapter 8 pp255)

This is a condition mainly in first litter gilts that may account for up to 3% increase in piglet mortality.

Symptoms

Sows

☞ Offending gilts can often be identified by their nervous apprehension at the onset of farrowing.

☞ They have a "wild eyed" look.

Causes / Contributing factors

- It is thought to be related, in part at least, to the major hormone changes that take place around parturition.

The following factors seem to predispose to it:

- A harsh or alien environment.
- Poor empathy between the gilts and the stockperson.
- Nutritional deficiencies.
- The effect of being placed in individual confinement for the first time.
- It may also be related to temperament.
- It seems to be more prevalent in some breeds than others.
- Alarming outbreaks have been experienced in new gilt herds where 100 - 150 pregnant animals have been reared together in straw yards. In such large groups no pecking order develops.

Diagnosis

Severe trauma to the skin and limbs. Clinical picture. History.

Treatment

❒ Try to identify potential gilts before farrowing.

❒ Watch each gilt during the birth of the first 2 or 3 piglets and if there is any sign of savaging, inject with azaperone (stresnil) at a dose level of 1ml/12kg weight. Confine all the piglets to the creep area for at least 20 minutes following injection until the gilt has settled down and rolled over on her side. The piglets should then be reintroduced. Most farrowings continue normally thereafter.

❒ Discuss with your veterinarian the possibility of treatment with mysoline. This drug is available in tablets containing 250mg of a drug called primidone which is an anti-convulsant drug but has the effect of reducing hysteria and nervousness. 3 to 4 tablets may be given twice daily 24 to 48 hours prior to farrowing.

Shoulder Sores

(Chapter 8 pp256)

They arise due to repeated bruising and pressure over the bony prominences on the shoulder blade. Ultimately the skin breaks, there is an erosion and a large sore develops. Such sows should not be kept for future breeding

Symptoms

Piglets

☞ N/A

Sows

☞ Highest point of the spine a reddening of the skin appears, which gradually forms into an ulcer.

☞ In severe cases the lesion may extend to 40 - 70mm in diameter with the development of extensive granulation tissue.

☞ Often both sides of the shoulder are affected.

Causes / Contributing factors

- They are associated with totally slatted flooring and individual sows that are too thin and have a prominent spine to the shoulder blade.
- First noticed in the farrowing crates where the floors are slippery.
- The sow has difficulty in rising, thus constantly bruising her shoulder.

Diagnosis

This is based on the clinical signs and ulcerating shoulders.

Treatment

❒ As soon as the condition appears move the sow into a well bedded pen. Feed ad lib for 2 to 4 weeks.

❒ Cut a hole slightly larger than the sore in a 70mm square piece of foam or thick carpet and place over the shoulder sore. Hold it in place with contact adhesive such as evostik. This pad will then protect the sore and allow it to heal.

❒ Watch for cannibalism by sucking pigs. If this occurs wean the sow.

❒ Large granuloma that sometimes develop can be surgically removed.

SPLAYLEGS

(Chapter 8 pp275)

This is a condition where the newborn piglet is unable to hold the front and/or (more commonly) back legs together and up to 2 % of piglets can be affected. The mobility of the piglet is impaired which makes teat access difficult.

Symptoms

Piglets

- ☞ The piglets are unable to stand with the hind legs deflected laterally.
- ☞ As a result they often adopt a dog sitting position.
- ☞ Death usually ensues either due to starvation or crushing because the pig cannot move away from the sow.

Causes / Contributing factors

- ◆ It is more common in the Landrace breed and in males.
- ◆ Disease is caused by immaturity of the muscle fibres in the hind legs, over the pelvis and occasionally in the front legs.
- ◆ The condition is exaggerated when piglets stand on very smooth or wet slippery floors.

Diagnosis

This is based upon the clinical signs.

Treatment

- ❒ As soon as the affected pig is identified use 25mm wide elasto-plast and tape the hind legs together leaving a gap of 50-80mm. The same procedure can be applied to the forelegs. The sticky tape should be passed around the legs just above the supernumer-ary digits. Never use string it will strangle the legs if not removed.
- ❒ Hold the piglet up by both its hind legs and vigorously massage the muscle masses over the pelvis and the front and rear of the hind legs. Repeat this 3 or 4 times during the first day.
- ❒ Assist the piglet to suckle regularly.
- ❒ Dose the pig with 10mls of sows colostrum or cows colostrum immediately after birth.
- ❒ Confine the strongest mobile pigs into the creep area for a period of one hour to allow splay leg pigs uninhibited access to the teats.

STILLBIRTHS

(Chapter 8 pp244)

When pigs are found dead behind the sow they are usually recorded as stillbirths which may be wrong. They may have died after farrowing having breathed but died of chilling and hypoglycaemia.

Symptoms

Piglets

☞ Found dead behind the sow. They may be fresh or 3 - 4 days old.

Causes / Contributing factors

- Stillbirths increase with the increasing age of the sow.
- Individual sows may be regular offenders and these can be identified by the sow litter card. The farrowing process should then be monitored.
- Stillbirths occur more in larger litters.
- Stillbirths are more common in pure breeds.
- Stillbirths are common in prolonged farrowings.
- Lack of exercise during pregnancy may raise stillbirth rates.
- Stillbirths are raised where there is a long gestation period.
- Farrowing house temperatures above 24°C (75°F) increase the risk of stillbirths.
- Uterine inertia results in stillbirths.
- High carbon monoxide levels in the air associated with faulty gas heaters can raise stillbirth rates significantly.
- Pigs found dead behind the sow can sometimes be related to particular farrowing crates in certain rooms and are due to draughts behind the sow.

An examination of records should clarify whether the problem is one of individual sows or across the herd.

Diseases of the sow which may result in stillbirths

- Anaemia.
- Aujeszky's disease.
- Eperythrozoonosis.
- Erysipelas.
- Leptospirosis.
- Mycotoxicosis.

- Parvovirus infection.
- PRRS.
- Toxoplasmosis.

Diagnosis

If the piglet dies before farrowing, it will show varying degrees of post mortem or degenerative changes. A pig that dies during the process of farrowing or immediately afterwards will be fresh and normal. The two can be differentiated easily. The chest is opened and the lungs examined to determine whether the pig had breathed. The lungs of the true stillborn pig are a dark plum colour, showing none of the pink areas associated with breathing. Pigs that attempt to breath during the process of farrowing will show evidence of mucous obstructing the wind pipe. A good target level for stillbirths is 3 to 5 % of total pigs born. At this level there is no point in carrying out investigations because it is unlikely that external inputs can alter the situation. However once the level reaches beyond 7% it is worthwhile carrying out an investigation by records and post-mortem examinations.

Streptococcal Meningitis

(Chapter 9 pp336)

Meningitis denotes inflammation of the meninges which are the membranes covering the brain. In the sucking piglet it is usually caused by *Streptococcus suis, Haemophilus parasuis,* or sometimes bacteria such as *E. coli* and other streptococci. *S. suis* has many serotypes. In most countries *S. suis* type 1 is the main one in sucking piglets, but this may not be true in other countries. For example in Denmark it is type 7. *S. suis* also causes joint problems particularly types 1 and 14.

S. suis is carried for long periods in the tonsils and may be transmitted to the sucking piglet from the sow or from other piglets. The sow also provides a variable level of immunity in the colostrum. Streptococcal meningitis in sucking piglets is sporadic in individual piglets. Streptococcal meningitis may be worse in sucking pigs when the organism has been introduced into the herd for the first time, or where it is secondary to infection with PRRS.

Symptoms

Sows

- ☞ Meningitis is uncommon.
- ☞ Muscle trembling.
- ☞ Head on one side.
- ☞ Nystagmus of the eyes.
- ☞ Incoordination.

Piglets / Weaners

- ☞ Symptoms of meningitis are rapid in onset.
- ☞ The piglet lying on its belly and shivering.
- ☞ It is characterised by a continual movement of the eyes from one side to the other (nystagmus).
- ☞ Paddling.
- ☞ Convulsions.
- ☞ In acute cases the piglet may be found dead.

Causes / Contributing factors

- *S. suis* is spread from one pig to another by direct nose to nose contact.
- Carrier boars or gilts.
- It can also spread within a herd by indirect contact.
- In confined space by aerosol infection.

Diagnosis

To confirm the diagnosis, the organism must be isolated from the meninges of clinically affected pigs and identified in a laboratory. The disease must be differentiated from joint infections, glässers disease, generalised septicaemia, salt poisoning, aujeszky's disease and hypoglycaemia.

Treatment

- ❒ If your herd has a problem examine the pigs twice daily to identify and treat affected pigs early.
- ❒ *Streptococcus suis* is usually sensitive to penicillin.
- ❒ Good nursing is equally important because the condition is very painful. Remove the piglet during the first 3 to 6 hours from the litter to a warm environment and carefully supplement it with milk via a stomach tube.

SUNBURN

This is a common condition in sows outdoors particularly in non pigmented breeds.

Ultra violet radiation not only damages the skin but also has an effect on the reproductive system and the maintenance of pregnancy.

Symptoms

Sows	Piglets
☞ Reddened skin.	Reddened skin.
☞ Blistering.	
☞ Wet dermatitis.	
☞ Pain.	
☞ Illness.	
☞ Reabsorption of embryos.	
☞ Irregular returns.	
☞ Abortions.	
☞ Will not accept boar at mating.	

Causes /Contributing factors

- Non pigmented breeding stock.
- Lack of shades.
- Lack of wallows.
- Poor maintenance of wallows.
- Brassica tops e.g. turnips, parsnips may predispose.

Diagnosis

This is by the clinical signs.

Treatment

- ❒ Remove badly affected pigs indoors.
- ❒ Apply barrier creams.
- ❒ Provide more wallows.

SWINE DYSENTERY (SD)

(Chapter 9 pp338)

Swine dysentery is caused by a bacterium called *Serpulina hyodysenteriae*. This organism causes a severe inflammation of the large intestine with a bloody mucous diarrhoea (i.e. dysentery).

Symptoms

Clinical disease in sows is uncommon unless new disease appears in the herd.

<u>All Pigs</u>

- ☞ Severe acute dysentery may occur.
- ☞ Sloppy light brown faeces with or without mucous or blood.
- ☞ Loss of condition.
- ☞ Sows become symptomless carriers.

Causes / Contributing factors

- It is a major disease in the growing pig but the breeding female can become a carrier for a long period of time and therefore acts as a potential source of infection to other pigs.
- Pigs become infected through the ingestion of infected faeces.
- It may enter the farm through the introduction of carrier pigs.
- Mechanically in infected faeces via equipment, contaminated delivery pipe of feed vehicles, boots or birds.
- It can be spread by flies, mice, birds and dogs.
- Stress resulting from change of feed may precipitate.
- Poor sanitation and wet pens enhance the disease.
- Overcrowding.

Diagnosis

This is by the clinical signs and laboratory identification of the organism.

Treatment

- ❐ By injection with lincomycin, tiamulin or tylosin.
- ❐ In-feed lincomycin, tiamulin, tylosin, carbadox, salinomycin.

Swine Fevers
African Swine Fever(ASF)
Classical Swine Fever(CSF) also known as Hog Cholera (HC)

(Chapter 12 pp403)

Swine fever is one of the most important virus diseases of pigs. It is notifiable inmost countries of the world. Control is by slaughter or as a last resort by vaccination. African swine fever (ASF) and Classical Swine fever are caused by very similar viruses which are only distinguishable by laboratory testing. Both are dealt with in *Chapter 12.*

Swine fevers are caused by one of the pesti family of viruses. The pig is the only natural host

The virus survives in frozen carcasses for long periods of time

Symptoms

<u>Piglets</u>

- ☞ Huddled.
- ☞ Chilled.
- ☞ Vomiting.
- ☞ Diarrhoea.
- ☞ Incoordination.
- ☞ Conjunctivitis.
- ☞ High fever.
- ☞ Death.

<u>Sows</u>

- ☞ When first introduced into the breeding herd include inappetence and high fevers.
- ☞ The virus can cross the placenta to invade the foetuses causing foetal death with mummification, abortions, malformations and increases in stillbirths.
- ☞ An important characteristic is the birth of very weak trembling piglets.
- ☞ Convulsions may occur with death within a few hours.
- ☞ Sows may lose the use of their legs.
- ☞ The disease in the acute form will have dramatic effects on reproduction.

Causes / Contributing factors

- The virus is spread from infected or carrier pigs via discharges from the nose, mouth and the urine and faeces and it is highly contagious.
- Infection enters the pig by the mouth by direct contact of one pig with another.
- It can get into herds by the introduction of infected meat.

- Mechanical spread via boots, clothing, lorries etc. is common.

Diagnosis

CSF is a rapid spreading disease with high mortality in all pigs. There are characteristic post-mortem changes with haemorrhagic lymph nodes, dead patches in the spleen, multiple small haemorrhages in the kidneys and so-called "button ulcers" in the gut.

These are all of diagnostic significance. Laboratory tests include the identification of viral antigen, isolation of the virus and the presence of antibodies in serum. In most countries CSF is notifiable.

Treatment

❒ There is no treatment.

The CSF virus is very persistent and survives in frozen tissues for long periods of time. In many countries there is a slaughter and eradication programme. Where there are widespread outbreaks of disease, vaccination is sometimes used to control the spread, followed often by slaughter policies.

Swine Influenza Virus (SI)

(Chapter 6 pp171)

Swine influenza is caused by a number of closely related influenza A viruses that are noted for their ability to change their antigenic structure and create new strains.

Each serotype is identified by surface proteins referred to as "H" and "N". The three common strains that affect the pig are described as $H_1 N_1$, $H_1 N_2$ and $H_3 N_2$. There are also different strains within these serotypes with differing pathogenicity (capacity to produce disease).

The incubation period of the disease is very short, as little as 12-48 hours.

There are three important periods when infection causes infertility. First, if sows are ill in the first 21 days post-service their developing embryos may not get established and an increase in 21 day returns results. If pregnancy has been established 14-16 days after mating, and it then fails, returns will be delayed. Second if infection occurs in the first five weeks of pregnancy, there could be total embryo mortality and absorption with sows becoming pseudo-pregnant and not in-pig. Litter size may also be affected at this stage due to absorption of embryos. Towards the end of the pregnancy period abortions or late mummified pigs at farrowing may also be experienced. The third major effect is on the boar, where high body temperatures affect semen and depress fertility for a 4 to 5 week period.

SI in large herds may become endemic with intermittent bouts of disease and infertility and different strains may also sequentially infect the herd. Immunity to influenza viruses is often short lived (6 months) and the immunity profile in the breeding herd varies considerably with time.

Symptoms

Piglets

- ☞ It would be unusual to see any signs of swine flu in the sucking pig unless disease entered the herd for the first time.
- ☞ Colostrum may prevent infection during the sucking period.
- ☞ Coughing.
- ☞ Pneumonia.
- ☞ Fever.

Sows

- ☞ High temperatures which cause abortions.
- ☞ Widespread coughing.
- ☞ Pneumonia

When the virus first enters the herd two or three animals may be observed sick for the first two days, followed by:

- ☞ A rapid explosive outbreak of inappetence and clinically very ill pigs.
- ☞ The effects on the reproductive system follow the sudden onset of a rapid spreading respiratory disease with coughing, pneumonia, fevers and inappetence.
- ☞ Acute respiratory distress persists over a period of 7-10 days (depending on the amount of contact between groups of sows).

At a herd level the following may also be seen:

- ☞ A sudden and rapid onset of acute illness in sows.

- ☞ Coughing and pneumonia spreading rapidly.
- ☞ A return to clinical normality over 7-10 days.
- ☞ Delayed returns to heat after weaning.
- ☞ Increased repeats at 21 days.
- ☞ Increased repeats outside the normal cycle.
- ☞ Increased numbers of sows coming through not in-pig.
- ☞ Increased numbers of abortions, particularly late term.
- ☞ Increased numbers of stillbirth rates and slow farrowings.
- ☞ Occasionally an increase in mummified pigs.
- ☞ During the phases of high temperatures other diseases present in the herd may be triggered off. A typical example would be an increase in abortions associated with leptospira infection.

Causes / Contributing factors

SI can be introduced by:

- Infected people.
- Carrier pigs.
- Probably on the wind although this has not been proved.
- Birds particularly water fowl, are reservoirs of infection.
- Secondary bacterial infections.
- Fluctuating temperatures.
- Stress.
- Wet bedding and floor surfaces.

Diagnosis

This can often be made reliably on clinical grounds with acute disease because there are no other diseases that are so dramatic in their onset and clinical effects. Blood samples taken at the time of onset of disease from affected sows and repeated 2-3 weeks later show rising levels of antibody to the specific virus. SIV can be readily grown from nasal and throat swabs and identified in the laboratory. This is often the best approach to confirm the diagnosis.

In acute disease the spread is so dramatic across all ages that little else can be confused with it. In endemic disease however differentiation from other viral infections can be difficult, but PRRS, PRCV, AD and also erysipelas should be considered.

Treatment

- ❐ Individual breeding females or boars showing acute illness, and raised temperatures, particularly with increased respiratory rate should be treated with broad spectrum antibiotics for three days.
- ❐ Suitable drugs would include penicillin/streptomycin, long-acting OTC or synthetic penicillins such as amoxycillin. If the illness is severe then medicate the drinking water with either CTC or OTC at a level of 25g (100% pure) per 1000kg of live weight per day, for five days.

Swine Pox

This is similar in all pigs see Section 3.

Swine Vesicular Disease (SVD)

This is similar in all pigs see Section 3.

Teat Necrosis

(Chapter 8 pp276)

Teat necrosis is a condition in which rubbing the end of the teat causes the teat tip to die (necrosis) and slough off. It is of no consequence in commercial herds which are buying in replacement gilts but it is very important where breeding females are being produced.

It first becomes evident 12 to 24 hours after birth. The teats in front of the umbilicus are the ones at risk because these have the greatest contact with the floor during sucking.

Commercially the condition is not important but it is if gilts are reared for breeding.

Symptoms

Piglets

- ☞ The teat end appears bright red gradually becoming black.
- ☞ The damage can be severe resulting in a blind or inverted teat.

Sows

- ☞ Teats may show permanent damage from trauma at birth.
- ☞ More common in the teats in front of the navel.

Causes / Contributing factors

- Trauma to the teats occurs on all floor surfaces but to a lesser extent on those that are well bedded with shavings or straw.

Diagnosis

Examine teats 8 - 24 hours after birth for red or black teat sphincters.

Treatment

❒ There is no treatment for this condition and prevention is necessary. The teats anterior to the umbilicus should be coated with a protective compound as soon as possible after birth. Use either elastoplast contact adhesive or cow gum.

TETANUS

(Chapter 8 pp277)

Tetanus is caused by the bacterium *Clostridium tetani* which produces toxins that affect the central nervous system. The organism, which can form spores, lives in the large intestines and faeces of many mammals and in certain soils. This disease can be a problem in outdoor pigs. The incubation period is from 1 to 10 weeks. It would be uncommon to see disease in the sucking piglet under 2 weeks of age.

Symptoms

<u>All Pigs</u>

☞ Hypersensitive.

☞ Shows stiffness of legs and muscles.

☞ An erect tail.

☞ Muscular spasms of the ears and face.

Causes / Contributing factors

- The bacteria must enter through a dirty abrasion or a cut.
- In the sucking pig the most common source is castration - unhygienic methods.

Diagnosis

This is based on the clinical symptoms.

Treatment

❒ Vaccination of the sow is highly effective.

Thin Sow Syndrome

(Chapter 7 pp222)

The thin sow syndrome develops over a period of months and one or two pregnancy cycles, with gradual declining body condition until 10 to 30% of the animals have a condition score of 1 or 2. During lactation the sow is unable to maintain her body condition due to an insufficient intake of energy combined with increasing milk output. This process continues over successive lactations.

In sows kept permanently outdoors the stockman should ensure that all the sows have a high body score before the start of cold weather.

Symptoms

Sows

☞ Thin emaciated sows.

☞ Body condition decreases with each successive pregnancy.

Piglets

☞ N/A

Causes / Contributing factors

The syndrome arises due to:

- Inadequate nutrition.
- Poor quality feeds.
- Damp floors or draughts will increase the energy requirement of the dry sow.
- Fluctuating temperatures.
- It is exacerbated in sows kept outdoors in cold weather.
- Heavy worm burdens.
- Specific diseases e.g. cystitis.

Diagnosis

This is by clinical signs. Select at least twelve faeces samples from thin sows. Submit them to a laboratory for examination to eliminate parasites and blood (from gastric ulcers). Eliminate specific individual diseases such as kidney infections and chronic infections.

Treatment

❒ Treatment should be aimed at increasing the nutritional intake of the sow during key periods of production.

❐ Raise feed intake across the whole herd by 1 to 2kg a day for a period of 10 to 14 days.

❐ Sows that have become very thin, should if possible, be moved from their dry sow accommodation and housed in warm deep straw pens in an environmental temperature of at least 20ºC (70ºF) and ad lib fed for 3 to 4 weeks using a lactating diet because the appetite in such animals is often depressed.

Thrombocytopaenic Purpura - Bleeding

(Chapter 8 pp277)

This is an uncommon condition seen only in young piglets from approximately 7 to 21 days of age. Disease commences 7 to 10 days after the intake of colostrum.

The piglet dies through the failure of normal blood clotting mechanisms. The disease is very sporadic but up to half the litter may be affected.

Symptoms

Piglets	Sows
☞ Clinical signs can be sudden.	☞ N/A
☞ Good pigs found dead.	
☞ Look closely at the skin of these and you will see haemorrhages wherever there has been bruising, teeth marks or trauma.	
☞ Haemorrhages are evident throughout all body tissues.	

Causes / Contributing factors

- It arises when the sows colostrum contains antibodies that destroy the piglets blood platelets (thrombocytes).
- The immune system of the sow during the period of pregnancy recognises the platelets as foreign protein and produces anti-bodies against them.
- The formation of these antibodies is also related to the boar that is used.

Diagnosis

Seek veterinary advice and post-mortem examinations. Can be confused with swine fever.

Treatment

- ❐ There is no treatment other than good nursing.
- ❐ Move the litter onto another sow.

Torsion of the Stomach and the Intestines

(Chapter 9 pp314)

Torsion of the stomach or the small intestine is a main cause of death in adult breeding stock. The twist can involve the stomach, the spleen, part of the liver or the intestine.

Symptoms

Sows	Piglets
☞ Bloated abdomen.	☞ Uncommon but symptoms as in sow.
☞ Sudden death.	

Causes / Contributing factors

- Overeating liquid feed.
- Excitement in anticipation of feeding.
- Abnormal carbohydrates and gassy fermentation in the small or large bowel.
- Large amounts of feed eaten during lactation will predispose.

Diagnosis

A post-mortem examination is necessary to confirm diagnosis.

Treatment

- ❐ None.
- ❐ Change feeding practices and feed constituents if the condition becomes a problem.

Transmissible-Gastro-Enteritis (TGE)

(Chapter 8 pp277)

TGE is a very important and highly infectious disease in the piglet caused by a coronavirus. The virus is killed by sunlight within a few hours but will survive for long periods outside the pig in cold conditions. It is very susceptible to disinfectants particularly iodine based ones, quaternary ammonia and peroxygen compounds.

Disease will persist in the farrowing houses over a period of 3 to

4 weeks until sows have developed sufficient immunity to protect the piglets.

In herds of less than 300 sows the virus is usually self eliminating provided there are good all-in, all-out procedures in farrowing houses and grower accommodation. In larger herds however the virus will persist in the growing herd because piglets at weaning, still under the influence of the maternal antibody, move into houses where the virus still persists. Once the lactogenic immunity in the sow's milk is no longer being taken in the pigs become infected allowing the virus to multiply. The pigs then shed the virus, contaminating the weaner rooms and infecting pigs being weaned after them. TGE can become endemic in herds in a mild form with high morbidity but low mortality.

Read *chapters 2 and 3* of the main manual on biological control of diseases entering the farm and the precautions necessary to prevent diseases spreading by faeces.

Symptoms

Piglets

☞ In the sucking piglet the disease is very severe.
☞ Acute watery diarrhoea.
☞ Almost 100% mortality within 2 to 3 days in piglets under 7 days of age due to severe dehydration and electrolyte imbalance.
☞ There is no response to antibiotic therapy.
☞ The most striking feature is the wet and dirty appearance of all the litter due to the profuse diarrhoea.

Sows

☞ In acute outbreaks the most striking feature is the rapidity of spread.
☞ Vomiting.
☞ Diarrhoea.
☞ Adult animals show varying degrees of inappetence and usually recover over a 5 to 7 day period.

Causes / Contributing factors

- The virus is shed in large numbers in the faeces.
- Pig faeces therefore are the major source of transmission either directly through the purchased carrier pig or indirectly through

mechanical transmission.

- Poor pen floors.
- Poor pen hygiene associated with bad drainage
- Poor hygiene procedures, between pens
- Environmental contamination from one pen to another i.e. boots, brushes, shovels clothing etc.
- Feeder pipes and feed bins. This is a high risk source for the spread of enteric diseases.
- Dogs may shed the virus in their faeces for 2 to 3 weeks.
- Birds and in particular starlings may transmit the disease.
- Contaminated feed.

Diagnosis

The clinical picture in acute disease is almost diagnostic. There are no other enteric diseases that spread so rapidly across all pigs. The ultimate diagnosis of TGE must be made in the laboratory from the intestine of a fresh dead pig using fluorescent antibody tests (FAT's). Isolation of the virus is also carried out.

Porcine epidemic diarrhoea (PED) could give a similar picture but it would be less acute and with less mortality in sucking pigs.

Treatment

- ❐ There is no specific treatment for TGE.
- ❐ Provide easy access to water containing electrolyte and an antibiotic such as neomycin.
- ❐ Improve the nursing and environment of the litter by providing extra heat and deep bedding to reduce the weights of infection from the diarrhoea.

Vice - Abnormal Behaviour

(Chapter 7 pp223)

Vice in the dry sow is confined to vulval biting particularly in the last 3 to 4 weeks of pregnancy. This can be a major problem in loose-housed sows and in badly managed systems there may be 80% of all sows in a herd with the vulva completely bitten off. Severely traumatised vulvas heal with scar tissue and this can cause constrictions and difficulties at farrowing.

Symptoms

Piglets

☞ N/A

Sows

☞ Lacerations of the vulva are common.

☞ Evidence of blood on the skin and noses of the sows highlight the possibility of this condition.

☞ Severe haemorrhage with loss of life in a few animals.

Causes / Contributing factors

- Vulval biting is much more common in pens that are long and narrow rather than those that are wide. There is less competition at feeding time in a wide pen.
- Vulva biting is also common when electronic feeder systems are used. It requires careful stockmanship and good pen design to prevent it.
- There is a relationship between vulva biting and feed intake, the size of the feed pellet, the type of floor surface and the bedding used. Many cases occur in the last 3 - 4 weeks of pregnancy.
- High stocking densities predispose.

Diagnosis

This is obvious from clinical evidence but an examination should be carried out to ensure the haemorrhage is not arising from the vagina, womb or bladder.

Treatment

❐ Because sows continue to traumatise an already damaged vulva it is most important that affected sows are removed from the group at the onset.

❐ In most cases once the sow is isolated the haemorrhage will stop and the tissues will shrink and heal.

❐ Occasionally it is necessary to stem the haemorrhage. To do this sedate or restrain the sow and apply a pressure using bandage as a tourniquet.

❐ If haemorrhage continues infiltrate local anaesthetic into the vulva and place two or more mattress sutures behind the bleeding points as described in *Chapter 15 pp 520* of the main manual.

Vitamin E Deficiency & Iron Toxicity

(Chapter 13 - pp428)

Iron toxicity occurs when the sow and her piglets are deficient in vitamin E. Iron dextran injections become toxic and cause severe muscle reactions at the injection site.

Symptoms

Piglets

☞ The piglets become acutely lame and the affected muscles swell.

☞ The piglets develop heavy breathing and look pale.

☞ Death occurs within 24 hours.

Sows

☞ None.

Causes / Contributing factors

- Vitamin E deficiency in the sow occurs when fats in the diet become rancid or cereals or corn have fermented and spoiled and the vitamin E is destroyed. Piglets are then born deficient
- Poor quality iron dextran will predispose.

Diagnosis

A history of acute lameness within 12 hours of iron injection, often with high mortality. Swellings at the sire of injection.

Treatment

❒ Inject sows due to farrow over the next 3 weeks with a vitamin E selenium preparation or water soluble vitamin E.

❒ Inject all litters for a 3 week period with vitamin E or dose by mouth at least 2 days before iron injections are given.

Vomiting and Wasting Disease / Ontario Encephalitis

(Chapter 8 pp279)

This is caused by a coronavirus which is widespread in the pig populations of North America and Europe but clinical disease is rare. This is because although the virus can infect susceptible pigs at any age it only causes clinical disease in newborn piglets. Most sows have been infected and are immune. They pass their immunity to their piglets in colostrum which protects them through the vulnerable period.

There is a variation in virulence between strains resulting in two different disease syndromes. Both start at around 4 days of age, are sudden in onset and affect whole litters

Symptoms

Sows

☞ N/A

Piglets

☞ Huddled.
☞ Hairy.
☞ Vomit bright green-yellow vomitus.
☞ Constipated.
☞ In the typical vomiting and wasting disease syndrome piglets lose their ability to suck or swallow, become very thirsty and stand with their heads over water but are unable to drink.
☞ They waste away, become severely emaciated and die.

In the typical encephalitis or brain infected syndrome they:

☞ Froth and champ at the mouth.
☞ Develop blueing of their extremities.
☞ Abdomens become bloated.
☞ Tremble.
☞ Stilted gait which rapidly progresses to partial paralysis of the legs.
☞ They lie down.
☞ Go into convulsions.
☞ Roll their eyes.
☞ Die within four days of onset.

Causes / Contributing factors

- Lack of immunity from sows to piglets via colostrum.

Diagnosis

The clinical and pathological picture is diagnostic of the disease. If you open up their abdomens you will find gas in the stomach and intestine but no food, only some brightly coloured liquid. You will also see brightly coloured crystals in the kidneys. A blood test is available.

Treatment

❒ There is no treatment and fortunately the disease will not occur again in this herd.

VULVAL HAEMATOMA

(Chapter 8 pp256)

This is a condition in which shortly after farrowing blood vessels inside the vulva rupture, due to stretching or trauma to the tissues. Always consider this as a serious condition that is life threatening. It requires frequent monitoring over 24 hours. It is often seen in gilts.

Symptoms

<u>Piglets</u>

☞ N/A

<u>Sows</u>

☞ The vulva fills with blood and becomes swollen and dark blue.

☞ When this occurs the tissues become very fragile and if they are crushed the vulva splits with severe haemorrhage which may not stop.

☞ The animal becomes anaemic and may bleed to death.

Causes / Contributing factors

- Trauma.
- Assisted farrowings.

Diagnosis

A blood filled vulva at farrowing.

Treatment

❒ The animal should be sedated using stresnil and local anaesthetic should be injected in the tissues nearest the body of the sow just forward of the bleeding area. Three methods are then used for control:

1. A piece of band or bandage is placed between the lips of the vulva and behind the bleeding tissues. It is then tightened to produce a tourniquet. This should be left for 24 hours.
2. If this does not stop the bleeding then a series of mattress sutures should be passed through the vulva and tied to the

exterior. See *chapter 15 pp 530* of the main manual.

3. If the haemorrhage still does not stop, the haematoma must be opened by a veterinarian who will use a pair of artery forceps to clamp the ruptured blood vessels and tie them off.

- ❒ Observe the effectiveness of the measures taken by placing a paper bag beneath the vulva so that any subsequent haemorrhage can be observed.
- ❒ Cover the tail gate of the crate with a bag of straw or other suitable protective material to stop further damage.

3

Recognising and Treating Disease in the Weaner, Grower and Finishing Herd

SECTION 3

RECOGNISING AND TREATING DISEASE IN THE WEANER, GROWER AND FINISHING HERD

Use the following table to identify the possible cause of disease based on your clinical observations:

Clinical signs	Causes / contributing factors
Abdomen distended (Blown up)	**Atresia ani** * - No rectum (newly weaned pigs) (Section 2) Chronic inflammation of the large intestine Constipation Fermentation in large intestine **Peritonitis** - (Section 2) **Prolapse of the rectum** **Rectal stricture** * Recto vaginal fistula **Torsion of the stomach and intestines** *
Abscesses	Fighting Generalised disease Poor injection technique **Tail biting** * **-** See **Vice** Trauma Wounds *
Anaemia	**Eperythrozoonosis** **Gastric ulcers**

Clinical signs	Causes / contributing factors
Arthritis	See **Lameness**
Blindness	**Botulism** Lead poisoning *(Chapter 13)* **Meningitis** (See **streptococcal infections**) **Salt poisoning (Water deprivation)**
Blisters	**Foot and mouth disease (FMD)** **Swine vesicular disease (SVD)** Other vesicular diseases *(Chapter 12)*
Blood from the/ on the nose	**Actinobacillus pleuropneumonia (App)** **Anthrax** **Atrophic rhinitis (AR) or (PAR)** * Poisonings e.g. warfarin *(Chapter 13)* Trauma *
Blood in faeces	Acute enteritis **Anthrax** **Clostridial diseases** **Coccidiosis** (occasionally) **Diarrhoea** **Gastric ulcers** Gut damage Haemorrhage **Parasites** **Porcine enteropathy (PE) - (bloody gut)** * **Swine dysentery (SD)** * Warfarin poisoning *(Chapter 13)*
Coughing	**Actinobacillus pleuropneumonia (App)** * Ammonia poisoning *(Chapter 13)*

Clinical signs	Causes / contributing factors
(Cont.)	**Aujeszky's disease (AD), (PR)** **Bordetellosis** Dust **Enzootic pneumonia (EP)** * **Glässers disease (Hps)** (recently weaned pigs) **Parasites,** Ascarids, Lungworm - out doors mainly *(Chapter 11)* **Pasteurellosis** **Porcine reproductive and respiratory syndrome (PRRS)** **Porcine respiratory corona virus (PRCV)** **Salmonellosis** **Swine influenza (SI)** *
Cuts and bruises	Fighting Trauma from the environment
Dehydration Sunken eyes, Loss of condition	Colitis **Diarrhoea** * **Fever** (Section 2) **Greasy pig disease** Haemorrhage Kidney failure **Pneumonia** **Rotavirus infection** * **Spirochaetal diarrhoea** **Swine dysentery (SD)** Toxic conditions **Transmissible gastro-enteritis (TGE)** * Vomiting Water shortage

Clinical signs	Causes / contributing factors
Diamond shaped lesions	**Erysipelas**
Diarrhoea, scour, enteritis	**Clostridial diseases** **Colitis** * **Cryptosporidiosis** (Section 2) **Diarrhoea** * - Coliform infections **Eperythrozoonosis (Epe)** **Parasites** Poor environment Poor nutrition *(Chapter 14)* **Porcine enteropathy (PE)** - Bloody gut **Porcine epidemic diarrhoea (PED**) **Porcine reproductive and respiratory syndrome (PRRS)** **Rectal stricture** **Rotavirus infection** * **Salmonellosis** **Spirochaetal diarrhoea** **Swine dysentery (SD)** * **Swine fevers** **Transmissible gastro-enteritis (TGE)** * **Yersinia infection**
Discharges from eyes	All respiratory diseases **Atrophic rhinitis (AR)** * **Pneumonia** **Porcine reproductive and respiratory syndrome (PRRS)** * **Swine fevers** Virus infections
Discharges from nose	**Actinobacillus pleuropneumonia (App)** **Atrophic rhinitis (AR)** *

Clinical signs	**Causes / contributing factors**
(Cont.)	**Bordetellosis** **Pasteurellosis** *
Discoloration of the skin Reddening, blueing (cyanosis)	**Abscesses** **Actinobacillus pleuropneumonia (App)** **Erysipelas** **Fever** (Section 2) Pasteurellosis Pericarditis Poor circulation **Porcine reproductive and respiratory syndrome (PRRS)** * **Porcine stress syndrome (PSS)** **Salmonellosis** * **(blue discoloration)** **Swine dysentery (SD)** **Swine fevers** * Toxic conditions *(Chapter 13)*
Dog sitting position	Fractured hip or long bones * Fractured spine * Muscle trauma Ruptured disc Spinal abscesses **Swine fevers** See also nervous symptoms
Fever - increased temperature (Section 2)	**Aujeszky's disease (AD)** Caused by certain viruses & bacteria **Dehydration** **Enzootic pneumonia (EP)** **Eperythrozoonosis (Epe)** **Glässers disease** Results from any generalised infection *

Clinical signs	Causes / contributing factors
(Cont.)	**Salmonellosis** **Swine fevers**
Fits - convulsions	See nervous signs
Fractures	**Electrocution** Fighting **Leg weakness, Osteochondrosis (OCD)** Nutritional inadequacies *(Chapter 14)* **Osteomalacia (OM)** Trauma * See also **Lameness**
Gangrene - (black smelling dead tissue)	See Section 2 - Sows
Greasy skin	Dead scurfy skin Excess oils in skin **Greasy pig disease** * Pityriasis *(Chapter 10)*
Grinding of teeth	**Gastric ulcers** Pain
Haemorrhage	See Section 2 - Sows
Hairiness	Chilling **Pneumonia** Scour (See **diarrhoea**) Shortage of essential fatty acids *(Chapter 14)* Sign of ill health *

Clinical signs	**Causes / contributing factors**
Head on one side or shaking	**Meningitis** (See **streptococcal infections)** **Middle ear infection** * See nervous signs
Heavy breathing	Heart problems Heat excess or heat stroke **Pneumonia** * **Swine influenza (SI)**
Incoordination	See nervous signs
Inflamed skin	Pustular dermatitis *(Chapter 10)* **Swine Pox**
Jaundice (yellow skin)	**Eperythrozoonosis (Epe)** **Leptospirosis** * Liver damage **Lymphosarcoma** Poisons *(Chapter 13)* **Salmonellosis**
Jerky eye movements (nystagmus)	**Meningitis** * (See **streptococcal infections**) **Salt poisoning (Water deprivation)** **Streptococcal infections**
Lameness (Abnormal movement)	**Actinobacillus pleuropneumonia (App)** **Arthritis** * **Back muscle necrosis** - growers (Sec. 2) **Bursitis (occasionally)** **Bush foot.** Claw damage **Erysipelas** Fighting

Clinical signs	Causes / contributing factors
(Cont.)	**Foot-and-mouth disease (FMD)** **Fractures** * **Glässers disease (Hps)** * High stocking densities **Leg weakness, Osteochondrosis (OCD)** * **Middle ear infection** (incoordination) **Mycoplasma arthritis** * **Oedema disease(OD)** - recently weaned pigs Poisoning *(Chapter 13)* Poor floor surfaces Poor nutrition *(Chapter 14)* **Porcine stress syndrome (PSS)** Rickets **Salt poisoning (Water deprivation)** **Streptococcal infections** **Swine fevers** **Swine vesicular disease (SVD)** **Tail biting - Abnormal behaviour** * Trauma - muscles, joints, bones *
Loss of leg function	**Fractures** Nervous or spinal damage
Meningitis	See **streptococcal infections**
Mortality	**Abscesses** **Actinobacillus pleuropneumonia (App)** * Acute or chronic enteritis **Anthrax** **Aujeszky's disease (AD)** **Clostridial diseases** **Diarrhoea** - Scour

Clinical signs	Causes / contributing factors
(Cont.)	**Electrocution** (Section 2) **Enzootic pneumonia (EP)** **Erysipelas** Fighting Gas poisoning *(Chapter 13)* **Gastric ulcers** **Glässers disease (Hps)** - recently weaned pigs **Greasy pig disease** **Leptospirosis** (rare) **Lymphosarcoma** **Meningitis** (See **streptococcal infections**) **Mulberry heart disease - Vitamin E deficiency** * **Oedema disease (OD) - Bowel oedema (EDEMA)** - recently weaned pigs **Pasteurellosis** Pericarditis Pleurisy **Pneumonia** * Poisons *(Chapter 13)* **Porcine enteropathy (PE)** * - Bloody gut in growers **Porcine stress syndrome (PSS)** - finishers **Prolapse of the rectum** Respiratory disease - see **pneumonia** **Salmonellosis** **Salt poisoning (Water deprivation)** **Streptococcal infections** Stress **Swine dysentery (SD)** **Swine fevers**

Clinical signs	Causes / contributing factors
(Cont.)	**Torsion of the stomach and intestines** * Toxic gasses *(Chapter 13)* Trauma **Vice - Abnormal behaviour** Whey bloat - growers
Mucus in faeces	**Colitis** **Diarrhoea** **Swine dysentery (SD)** *
Mucus, pus in the urine	**Cystitis** (bladder infection) - Section 2 **Pyelonephritis** (kidney infection) - Sec. 2
Muscle trembling	See Section 2 - Sows
Nervous signs For e.g. Trembling of muscles Incoordination Lameness Meningitis Paraplegic Brain infection	Abscess spine **Aujeszky's disease** (AD), (PR) **Classical swine fever (CSF)** **(Hog cholera)** **Glässers disease (Hps)** **Middle ear infection** **Mycoplasma arthritis** **Oedema disease** (OD) - recently weaned pigs Poisoning *(Chapter 13)* **Salmonellosis** **Salt poisoning (Water deprivation)*** **Streptococcal infections** * Talfan, Teschen disease - weaners Tetanus
Not eating (inappetence)	**Diarrhoea** **Fever** (Section 2)

Clinical signs	Causes / contributing factors
Temperature elevated (Cont.)	**Glässers disease** **Lameness** Many infectious diseases (e.g. **Erysipelas, Influenza, PRRS)** **Pneumonia** * **Salmonellosis** Septicaemia * **Swine fevers**
Not eating (Inappetence) Temperature normal	**Atrophic rhinitis (AR)** Bullying Diarrhoea **Gastric ulcers** Gastritis **Lameness** **Oedema disease - bowel oedema** Poisoning *(Chapter 13)* **Porcine reproductive and respiratory syndrome (PRRS)** * **Salt poisoning - Water deprivation** Stomach ulcers **Swine dysentery (SD)** Twisted gut Unpalatable food Water shortage
Pain	**Arthritis** **Fractures** **Meningitis** (See **streptococcal infections**) **Oedema disease (OD)** Bowel oedema (EDEMA) **Torsion of the stomach and intestines** **Rectal stricture**

Clinical signs	Causes / contributing factors
Pale pigs	**Actinobacillus pleuropneumonia (App)** **Anaemia** * (Section 2) **Eperythrozoonosis (Epe)** **Gastric ulcers** Haemorrhage * **Leptospirosis** **Lymphosarcoma** **Mulberry heart disease** **Parasites** **Porcine enteropathy (PE)** - Bloody gut - growers **Prolapse of the rectum** Shortage of iron *
Paralysis	See **Lameness**
Pimples and/or small bite marks	Pustular dermatitis * Septicaemia **Swine pox** Trauma
Pneumonia / Heavy breathing	**Actinobacillus pleuropneumonia (App)** * **Aujeszky's disease (AD)**, (PR) **Enzootic pneumonia (EP)** **Eperythrozoonosis (Epe)** **Glässers disease (Hps)** **Parasites** **Pasteurellosis** **Porcine reproductive and respiratory syndrome (PRRS)** **Salmonellosis** **Streptococcal infections**

Clinical signs	Causes / contributing factors
(Cont.)	**Swine influenza (SI)**
Poor doing pigs, wasting, hairy	**Actinobacillus pleuropneumonia (App** Chronic enteritis **Diarrhoea** Draughts **Enteric diseases** * **Eperythrozoonosis (Epe)** **Glässers disease** * Low temperature Malabsorption Poor environment Poor nutrition (Chapter 14) **Porcine enteropathy (PE)** **Porcine reproductive and respiratory syndrome (PRRS)** * **Rectal stricture** Respiratory disease - see **pneumonia** **Salmonellosis** **Salt poisoning - (Water deprivation)** Shortage of water **Swine influenza (SI)** Villus atrophy
Prolapse of rectum	Excess gas in the bowel Increased abdominal pressure Nutritional factors *(Chapter 14)* Prolonged lying on a slope Rectal damage at mating Shortage of water
Rubbing / scratching	Harvest mites Mange *, Lice *(Chapter 11)*

Clinical signs	Causes / contributing factors
Salivation	**Foot and mouth disease (FMD)** **Swine vesicular disease (SVD)** Trauma
Skin diseases / conditions	Ear biting **Erysipelas** * Flank biting * **Foot and mouth disease(FMD)** **Greasy pig disease** * Lice *(Chapter 11)* Mange * Nutritional deficiencies *(Chapter 14)* Penis sucking - **Vice** Pityriasis rosea *(Chapter 10)* Poisons - warfarin *(Chapter 13)* **Porcine reproductive and respiratory syndrome (PRRS)** * Purpura - bleeding Ringworm *(Chapter 10)* **Salmonellosis** (blue colouration) **Swine pox** (round black lesions) **Swine fevers** **Swine vesicular disease (SVD)** Tail biting * - **Vice** **Vice** (abnormal behaviour)
Sneezing	Ammonia poisoning *(Chapter 13)* **Atrophic rhinitis (AR)** *, (PAR) **Aujeszky's disease (AD)** **Bordetellosis** Dust * Poor environment **Porcine cytomegalovirus infection**

Clinical signs	Causes / contributing factors
(Cont.)	**(PCMV)** * (Section 2) **Porcine reproductive and respiratory syndrome (PRRS)** Virus infections
Starvation - wasting	Actinobacillus pleuropneumonia (App) Chronic diseases *- respiratory / enteric **Gastric ulcers** **Glässers disease (Hps)** Malabsorption in weaners **Pasteurellosis** Pericarditis **Porcine enteropathy (PE)** - Bloody gut
Swellings of joints, muscles, tendons and others	**Abscesses** **Arthritis** * Arthritis caused by a septicaemia (Bacterial invasion of the body) **Bursitis** **Clostridial diseases** **Erysipelas** * **Fractures** **Haematoma** **Lameness** **Leg weakness, Osteochondrosis (OCD)** **Mycoplasma arthritis** * **Ruptures or hernias** Trauma See also **Lameness**
Trembling	**Porcine stress syndrome (PSS)** **Salt poisoning (Water deprivation)** See nervous signs

Clinical signs	Causes / contributing factors
Ulceration of the skin	**Bush foot / Foot rot** Dermatitis Granuloma (see **Bursitis**) Open wounds Pustular dermatitis *(Chapter 10)* Trauma Vesicular diseases (**FMD, SVD**)
Urine colour abnormal	(Chalky mineral deposits or abnormal colour) **Cystitis / pyelonephritis -** (Sec. 2)
Vice (Abnormal behaviour) e.g tail biting, ear biting, penis sucking, navel sucking.	Draughts Fluctuating temperatures **Greasy pig disease** High ammonia and carbon dioxide levels High stocking densities Mixing pigs Poor environment Poor feeding systems Poor nutrition *(Chapter 14)* Uncomfortable pigs
Vomiting	Coughing **Fever** (Section 2) **Fungal poisoning** (Section 2) **Gastric ulcers** Gastritis Poisoning (Chapter 13) **Porcine epidemic diarrhoea (PED)** **Transmissible gastro-enteritis (TGE)** **Vomiting and wasting disease** (Sec. 2)

*** More likely**

ABSCESSES

(See Chapter 7 pp199)

Abscesses are pockets of pus that contain dead cell material and large numbers of bacteria.

Symptoms

- ☞ Swellings.
- ☞ Evidence of fluid - pus or blood in swelling.
- ☞ Red skin.
- ☞ Often damage in skin.

Causes/Contributing factors

- ◆ Fighting and trauma.
- ◆ Secondary infection following tail biting.
- ◆ Small widespread abscesses in the skin (pustular dermatitis) may be seen following general illness, septicaemia and/or greasy pig disease.
- ◆ Damage to the skin by sharp objects in the environment.
- ◆ Poor injections.
- ◆ Chronic abscesses may form around joints following fractures.

Diagnosis

Feel and press the swelling to ascertain if the contents are fluid or solid. Sample the contents by inserting an 18mm 16 gauge needle attached to a 10ml syringe at the lowest soft point of the swelling.

Haemorrhage into the tissues is the only condition likely to be confused with an abscess. In such cases either pure blood or a very thin blood stained liquid will be withdrawn. Such pockets of blood are called haematomas.

Treatment

- ❒ Test the contents with a needle and syringe - blood or pus.
- ❒ Drain the pus by making an incision with a sharp scalpel blade approximately 15-20mm long at the lowest point particularly where it feels soft. Sometimes drainage will occur spontaneously after the abscess bursts.
- ❒ Squeeze into the hole an antibiotic cream (a cow mastitis tube is ideal) containing penicillin/streptomycin, oxytetracycline, amoxycillin or ampicillin or give an intramuscular injection of penicillin.

- ❒ Tail bitten pigs should be removed immediately from the pen and given a long-acting penicillin or OTC injection. Such pigs should not be sent for slaughter until the abscess has been lanced and drained as described in *Chapter 15 pp 495* and antibiotic withdrawal periods have been satisfied.
- ❒ For others address the causal problem.

Actinobacillus Pleuropneumonia (App)

(See Chapter 9 pp299)

The bacterium *Actinobacillus pleuropneumoniae* (App) consists of at least twelve different serotypes, some of which produce no disease but others cause severe disease. Serotypes vary in different countries. Types 1, 5, 9, 11 and 12 are usually highly virulent and strains 3 and 6 are mild. App is carried in the tonsils and upper respiratory tract. It is transmitted short distances by droplet infection and only survives outside the pig for a few days.

The organism may affect the pig from weaning through to slaughter but usually the age is from 8 to 16 weeks. The incubation period is very short, as little as 12 hours. Toxins produced severely damage the lungs.

App is uncommon in sows unless they are naive or disease is triggered by PRRS or flu.

Symptoms

- ☞ Sudden death/mortality - only sign a bloody discharge from the nose.
- ☞ Sudden death/mortality - no symptoms and more than 1 % of such deaths.
- ☞ A short cough perhaps 1 to 3 coughs at a time - different from the prolonged coughing of EP.
- ☞ Severe breathing difficulties.
- ☞ Blueing of the ears.
- ☞ Badly affected pigs are:
  - Severely depressed.
  - Body temperatures are high.
- ☞ Pleurisy.

☞ Haemorrhage from the nose.
☞ Lameness.
☞ Pale pigs.
☞ Pneumonia.
☞ Poor pigs - wasting and hairy.

Causes / Contributing factors

- Contaminated or carrier incoming pigs.
- Can be spread mechanically by equipment and visitors.
- Water deprivation.
- Low temperature and low humidity predisposes.
- Stress / movement.
- Nutritional changes.
- Continual production.

Diagnosis

This is based on herd history, clinical signs, post-mortem examinations including slaughter house checks and culture of the organism in the laboratory. The lesions in the lung are very characteristic. Serology can be used to identify different serotypes but the interpretation can be difficult because of cross reactions between serotypes.

App must be differentiated from enzootic pneumonia, PRRS, flu, and *Salmonella choleraesuis* pneumonia.

Treatment

❒ In view of the acute course of the disease it is important to identify clinical cases very early and treat individuals by injection. Affected pigs stop eating or drinking so that water or feed medication is usually ineffective. App usually has a wide range of antibiotic sensitivities. On the first day inject the pig twice eight hours apart. The following antibiotics are usually effective.
- Amoxycillin.
- Ampicillin.
- Ceftiofur. This is a very rapid acting drug and gives a good response.
- Enrofloxacin.
- OTC, LA. This can be used in more chronic cases. Repeat every two days.

- Penicillin.
- Penicillin/streptomycin.

❒ Determine when the onset of the disease is likely to occur and apply strategic medication just prior to this time.

❒ In-feed medication during the period of risk include:
- Phenoxymethyl penicillin 200-400g/tonne.
- Chlortetracycline 500-800g/tonne.
- Trimethoprim/sulpha 300-400g/tonne.
- Oxytetracycline 500-800g/tonne.

Preventive feed medication is not always effective probably because of the rapid onset of disease and rapid loss of appetite.

❒ Water medication during the period of risk can be more effective in preventing disease. Treat for 4-7 days. Similar drugs to in-feed medication can be used.

❒ In an acute outbreak examine the at risk group three times daily to identify disease as early as possible. It may be necessary to inject or water medicate the whole group. The decision to inject is a balance between effect, and risk of more disease due to the stress of handling the pigs.

❒ Vaccines are available.

Anaemia

This is similar in all pigs - see Section 2.

Anthrax

(See Chapter 9 pp301)

This disease is rare in the growing pig unless contaminated food has been purchased. The disease is transmissible to people. Effective vaccines are available in some countries for both pigs and people.

Symptoms

☞ Sudden death with no signs (or with swollen discoloured necks) and more than 1%.

☞ Bloody faeces.

☞ Haemorrhage from the nose.

Causes / Contributing factors

- Contaminated feed or water.

Diagnosis

Anthrax should be suspected if a pig is found dead and post-mortem examination shows copious blood tinged tissue fluid and large red lymph nodes under the skin of the neck and in the abdomen. The post-mortem examination should be discontinued immediately and veterinary help sought.

Treatment

❒ Penicillin is effective.

❒ Vaccines are available.

ARTHRITIS - JOINT INFECTIONS

(See Chapter 9 pp317)

Arthritis is inflammation of one or more joints and is common in the growing pig.

Symptoms

☞ Lameness, Swollen joints.

☞ Reluctance to stand.

☞ May be signs of specific disease.

Causes / Contributing factors

(* common)

- Brucellosis (in countries where this exists).
- Glässers disease (*Haemophilus parasuis*). *
- Erysipelas.*
- Mycoplasma arthritis (*Mycoplasma hyosynoviae* infection). *
- Leg weakness, Osteochondrosis (OCD) .*
- Streptococcal infection .*
- Trauma. *

Diagnosis

In many cases the only clinical sign is lameness. If a problem exists it is necessary to identify the organisms or diseases responsible, by post-mortem or bacteriological examinations.

Treatment

❒ Specific treatment will depend on the cause.

❐ Use penicillin by injection. There is a good response to erysipelas within 24 hours. There is no response to mycoplasma infection.

❐ Use Lincomycin or tiamulin. If mycoplasma are the cause a response will be seen in 24 - 48 hours.

Atrophic Rhinitis (AR) - Progressive Atrophic Rhinitis (PAR)

(Chapter 9 pp301)

Rhinitis, inflammation of the nose, can be caused by a variety of bacteria, viruses and irritant substances. During the process of infection the delicate turbinate bones in the nose become damaged and may shrink (atrophy). Progressive atrophic rhinitis describes a specific disease in which the turbinates atrophy permanently. It is caused by toxin producing strains of the bacteria *Pasteurella multocidia*. Infection is usually picked up after weaning, following which clinical disease may become evident. Sows are often carriers of *Pasteurella multocidia*

Symptoms

☞ Early signs can be seen in sucking pigs; sneezing, snuffling and a nasal discharge.

☞ Sneezing often blood stained.

☞ Tear staining and twisting, shortening and wrinkling of the nose.

☞ Reduced daily gain and variable growth.

☞ Reduced feed efficiency.

☞ Difficulty eating.

☞ Increase in respiratory diseases.

Causes / Contributing factors

- Spread of disease between herds is mainly by the carrier pig.
- Spread within herds is by droplet infection between pigs or by direct nose to nose contact.
- Spread indirectly on equipment, clothes etc.
- Poor environments and nutrition increase the severity.

Milder rhinitis, in the absence of toxigenic pasteurella (non progressive disease) in which the turbinate bones heal and regenerate, may be caused by the following.

- Air containing high bacterial counts.
- Aujeszky's disease (pseudorabies).
- *Bordetella bronchiseptica* infection.
- Chronic respiratory disease.
- Dust.
- Glässers disease.
- High levels of ammonia.
- Porcine cytomegalovirus infection (including body rhinitis).
- Porcine reproductive and respiratory syndrome (PRRS).
- Poor humid conditions.

Diagnosis

This is based on clinical signs. However do not assume if sneezing alone is occurring in young pigs that it will necessarily lead to progressive atrophic rhinitis. The disease is easily identified by post-mortem examinations of the nose and culture of the organism from nasal swabs. (See *Chapter 15 pp521* for information on swabbing).

Treatment

In acute outbreaks

- ❒ All adult stock should be vaccinated twice 4 to 6 weeks apart. Modern vaccines are very efficient.
- ❒ Sows should then be vaccinated prior to each farrowing.
- ❒ All weaned pigs should be medicated in-feed until the clinical outbreak has subsided.
- ❒ Antibiotic treatment should be given to the piglets. Apply the following :
  - Days 3 and 10 of age and at weaning, inject with either long-acting OTC or amoxycillin.
  - For three weeks post-weaning the creep feed should be med icated with OTC or CTC at dose levels of 500-800g/tonne or trimethoprim/sulpha (TMS).
  - Other antibiotics could be used depending on the bacterial sensitivity.
- ❒ The sows feed should be top-dressed with either OTC or

trimethoprim/sulpha (TMS) commencing five to seven days prior to farrowing and throughout the farrowing period, or the lactating ration medicated with trimethoprim/sulpha (500g).

Vaccination of the sows usually prevents infection up to about 10 weeks of age until the pigs move into finishing houses. Then, unless the grower house has been depopulated, the pigs will become infected but with mild clinical signs. Infection however increases the predisposition to other respiratory diseases and depresses feed intake and performance.

PAR may be eradicated from the herd after a 12 month period of sow vaccination provided all clinical evidence of disease has subsided. *(See Chapter 3 pp 94)*

Aujeszky's Disease (AD) / Pseudorabies (PR)

(Chapter 12 pp396)

This important disease is caused by a herpes virus. The pig is the main host. It can affect other species which do not spread it, including cattle, horses, dogs and cats. They all die. There are no confirmed reports of it affecting people. The virus can remain hidden in nerves of the pig in a carrier state for long periods of time and then be reactivated.

Symptoms

- ☞ Fever.
- ☞ Sneezing.
- ☞ Coughing.
- ☞ Pneumonia.
- ☞ Nervous signs including incoordination and fits.
- ☞ Some strains of the virus can cause severe respiratory disease and others severe rhinitis.
- ☞ Usually low mortality.

Causes / Contributing factors

- Field virus can be spread between herds by sub-clinical carrier pigs and on the wind.
- Wind-borne infection can occur over distances of several kilo-

metres over land and much further over water.

- The virus can be spread by AI.
- Within herds it may be spread by nose to nose contact, or by aerosol droplets.
- Periods of stress may activate disease.
- Continual production systems perpetuate disease.

Diagnosis

This is based on the clinical picture, serological and laboratory tests.

Treatment

- There is no specific treatment for AD.
- In-feed antibiotics may help to control secondary bacterial infections during the exposure to the virus.
- Eradication polices range from slaughter and repopulation, to a combination of vaccination and serology. Because the disease is relatively slow spreading it can be eliminated through vaccination, good management control and elimination of carriers.
- Vaccination should be carried out both in the face of acute disease and in control.

Back Muscle Necrosis

This is similar in all pigs - see Section 2.

Bloody Gut

See **Porcine Enteropathy.**

Bordetellosis

(See Chapter 9 pp304)

Bordetella bronchiseptica is a bacterium found in most if not all pig populations. Some strains cause a mild and non progressive rhinitis that heals spontaneously. The disease is clinically and economically of no consequence. However if toxigenic pasteurella are present in the herd then a combination of the two organisms can produce severe progressive rhinitis (PAR).

Bordetella bronchiseptica can also be a secondary opportunist invader in pneumonia.

Symptoms

- ☞ Coughing.
- ☞ Sneezing.
- ☞ Nasal discharge.

Causes / Contributing factors

- High levels of the bacteria may predominate in poor environments.
- Recirculation of air in nurseries allows a build up of organisms.
- Continual use of housing.

Diagnosis

This is based on cultural and laboratory examinations.

Treatment

- ❒ None needed unless levels are high.
- ❒ In-feed medicate with trimethoprim sulpha or chlortetracycline.
- ❒ Inject weaners with oxytetracycline long acting at weaning.

BOTULISM

This is similar in all pigs see Section 2.

BRUCELLOSIS

This is similar in all pigs see Section 2.

BURSITIS

(See Chapter 9 pp304)

Bursitis is a common condition that arises from constant pressure and trauma to the skin overlying any bony prominence. The membrane covering the bone reacts by creating more bone, a swelling develops and the skin becomes thicker until there is a prominent soft lump. Bursitis may cause the skin to become broken and secondary infection can develop. Mycoplasma can also infect the fluid in the swelling.

It can start in the farrowing houses, particularly if there are bad floors but it usually starts in the weaner accommodation on slatted floors which have large gaps. As the pig increases in weight there is increased pressure on the leg bones. Under normal circumstances, if there is no secondary infection, the condition is not commercially important but if breeding stock is being produced then the system needs to be adjusted or there will be a drop in selection rates.

Symptoms

- ☞ Swellings develop over the lateral sides of the hocks and elbows and over the points of the hocks.
- ☞ Occasional lameness may be seen.

Causes / Contributing factors

- ◆ Floor type - Wire mesh, woven metal and metal bar floors can produce high levels in weaner pigs in first and second stage housing.
- ◆ Concrete slats cause problems.
- ◆ Leg weakness may predispose.
- ◆ It can start in sucking pigs on slatted floors.

Diagnosis

Visual examination.

Treatment

- ❒ There is no specific treatment.
- ❒ If the swellings have become infected with bacteria inject with either oxytetracycline or ampicillin.
- ❒ If *Mycoplasma hyosynoviae* is causing infection use either lincomycin or tiamulin.
- ❒ Remove pigs to well bedded pens.
- ❒ Determine the point at which lesions are occurring and review environment.

Bush Foot / Foot Rot

(See Chapter 9 pp304)

Bush foot results from infection of the claw which becomes swollen and extremely painful around the coronary band. It usually occurs in one foot only and is more commonly seen in the hind feet especially the outer claws, which are the larger ones carrying proportionately more weight. Infection sometimes penetrates the soft tissues between the claws and this is referred to as foot rot. Foot rot involves both superficial and deep infection of the soft tissues between the claws often caused by fusiform bacteria.

Invariably, unless foot rot has developed, only one claw is involved.

Symptoms

☞ Lameness.

☞ Painful swollen claw.

☞ Cracks at the sole-hoof junction, or splitting of the hoof itself.

☞ As the infection progresses inside the hoof, the claw becomes enlarged and infection and inflammation of the joint often develops.

☞ In most cases a swelling is visible around the coronary band which may form an abscess and burst to the surface.

Causes / Contributing factors

- It arises through penetration of the sole of the foot.
- Cracks at the sole-hoof junction, or splitting of the hoof itself predispose.
- Poor concrete surfaces with sharp aggregate cause damage.
- Biotin deficiency predisposes.

Diagnosis

This is based on the clinical signs. Bush foot has to be differentiated from other forms of trauma and infection including erysipelas, glässers disease, leg weakness or osteochondrosis (OCD) and mycoplasma arthritis.

Treatment

Examine the feet when the animal is lying down.

❐ There will be a poor blood supply to the infected tissues and therefore higher dose levels of antibiotics are required for longer periods of time.

❐ Antibiotics which can be used include:

- Lincocin 11mg/kg liveweight.
- Oxytetracycline 25 mg/kg liveweight.
- Amoxycillin 15mg/kg liveweight.

❐ Inject daily for 5 to 7 days.

If there is no improvement in three days change the antibiotic.

Complete recovery may take 3-4 weeks.

❐ An anti-inflammatory drug such as phenylbutazone may be

administered either by mouth or injection.

- ❐ If there is a herd problem a foot bath containing either 1% formalin (only use in the open air) or 5% copper sulphate will help. Walk the sows through once each week on 2-3 occasions. However if there are dry cracked claws in the herd, this treatment might make them worse.
- ❐ Check the biotin levels in the diet.

Clostridial Diseases

(See Chapter 7 pp203)

Clostridial infections are relatively uncommon in growers and finishers. Section 2 has additional information.

Symptoms

- ☞ Sudden death in well grown.
- ☞ Haemorrhage - faeces.
- ☞ Diarrhoea.
- ☞ Painful and discoloured swellings over muscle masses.
- ☞ Gangrene.

Causes / Contributing factors

- Damage to the skin allowing bacteria to enter.
- High numbers of bacteria in the environment.

Diagnosis and Treatment

Post mortem examinations should be carried out as soon as possible. Anthrax should also be considered as a possibility. See section 2 for further information.

Coccidiosis (Coccidia)

(See Chapter 11 pp379)

This is a disease of sucking pigs but is seen occasionally in growing and finishing pigs and boars when they are moved or housed into continually populated and infected pens.

Symptoms

- ☞ Poor growth.
- ☞ Sloppy faeces.
- ☞ Faeces may occasionally be tinged with blood.

Causes / Contributing factors

- Dirty pens.
- Continual use of pens.
- Recycling of faeces.

Diagnosis

Examine faeces samples for the presence of the egg forms of the parasite. Only high numbers > 20,000 suggest disease.

Treatment

- ❒ Sulphonamides: Inject every other day for three applications or medicate the drinking water for seven days.
- ❒ Depopulating and washing out the pen using a disinfectant such as OO-CIDE will remove the coccidial oocysts.
- ❒ In adults the disease is usually self eliminating.

COLITIS

"Colitis" means inflammation of the large bowel. It is common in some countries in growing pigs and is characterised by diarrhoea. It is uncommon in home milled cereal based diets.

Affected pigs are usually 6 to 14 weeks of age and in any one group, up to 50% may be affected. It is not seen in adult or sucking pigs. Colitis may be seen in individual sows. A number of organisms have been implicated but *Serpulina pilosicoli*, an organism distinct from the one that causes swine dysentery, is thought to be important.

Symptoms

- ☞ Usually appear in rapidly growing pigs from 6 to 14 weeks old fed ad lib on high density diets.

The early signs:

- ☞ Sloppy "cow pat" type faeces, with no blood and little if any mucus.
- ☞ Pigs appearing otherwise normal.

As the disease and its severity progress:

- ☞ Watery diarrhoea.
- ☞ Dehydration.
- ☞ Loss of condition.
- ☞ Poor growth.

During the affected period:

- ☞ Daily gain and food conversion can be severely affected, with feed conversion worsening by up to 0.2.
- ☞ Mortality is low but morbidity can be high, ranging from 5 to 50%.

Causes / Contributing factors

- Dietary factors. Disease is experienced using all types of diets but particularly those that have been pelleted rather than fed as a meal. It is thought that the pelleting process may have an effect on fats in the diet and thereby initiate digestive disturbances in the large bowel.
- It is more common with diets high in energy and protein (14.5MJ DE/kg 21% protein).
- Certain components in the feed may also be implicated.
- It is common when fat sprayed diets are fed.
- Continual production predisposes.

Diagnosis

This is based on clinical signs and the elimination of other causes of diarrhoea, in particular swine dysentery. Faecal examinations in the laboratory are necessary to assist with diagnosis together with post-mortem examinations and laboratory tests on a typical untreated pig. It is possible that porcine enteropathy may be involved.

Treatment

- ❒ Antibiotic therapy is not always successful because it depends on the presence of primary or secondary bacteria, but the following drugs have given responses on problem farms, using in-feed medication.

Dimetridazole	- 200 g / tonne if available
Lincomycin	- 110 g/ tonne
Monensin	- 100 g / tonne if available
Oxytetracycline	- 400 g / tonne
Salinomycin	- 60 g / tonne
Tiamulin	- 100 g / tonne
Tylosin	- 100 g / tonne

- ❒ For the individual pig daily injections of either tiamulin, lincomycin, tylosin or oxytetracycline may be beneficial

CRYPTOSPORIDIOSIS

This is similar in all pigs see Section 2.

CYSTITIS AND PYELONEPHRITIS

This is similar in all pigs see Section 2.

DIARRHOEA OR SCOUR

(See Chapter 9 pp306 and pp308)

The bacterium *E. coli* is a common cause of diarrhoea. At weaning the loss of sow's milk and secretory IgA allows the *E. coli* to attach to the villi of the small intestines, the toxins produced then cause acute diarrhoea, usually within five days of weaning.

Symptoms

- ☞ The first signs are often slight loss of condition, dehydration and a watery diarrhoea.
- ☞ In some cases blood or black tarry faeces may be seen or they may be like paste with a wide range of colour: grey, white, yellow and green. The colour is not significant.
- ☞ Poor pigs - wasting, hairy.
- ☞ Sloppy faeces and often dirty wet pens.
- ☞ Sunken eyes.
- ☞ Dehydration results in rapid loss of weight.
- ☞ Pigs may be found dead with sunken eyes and slight blueing of the extremities.
- ☞ Good pigs may also be just found dead with no external symptoms.

Causes / Contributing factors

- ◆ Pre-weaning
  - Are the weaning problems mainly in gilt litters? If so consider *E. coli* vaccination in gilts.
  - Creep feeding. Consider the type, frequency and age of introduction.
  - Stop creep feeding before weaning and assess the effects.
- ◆ At weaning consider:
  - Stress.
  - Stocking density - group sizes.

- House temperatures and temperature fluctuations.
- Poor house hygiene.
- Continually populated houses.
- Water shortage.
- Feed type
  - Meal or pellets, wet or dry.
  - Feeding practices.
  - Quality of nutrition.

- After weaning consider the effects of:
  - Air flow - chilling.
  - Temperature fluctuations.
  - High ventilation and humidity.
  - Creep feed management.
  - Assess the response to different creep diets.
  - Consider other diseases present.
  - Age and weight at weaning.
  - Floor surfaces - provide comfort boards.
  - Asses rate and evenness of growth.

A diarrhoea problem in growing pigs is likely to be associated with one or more of the following diseases.
(Most common *):

- Classical swine fever (in those countries where it is still endemic).
- Coliform infections. *
- Colitis (non specific). *
- Parasites.
- Porcine epidemic diarrhoea (PED). *
- Porcine enteropathy including PIA, NE and RI. *
- Rotavirus infection.
- Salmonellosis. *
- Spirochaetal diarrhoea.
- Swine dysentery. *
- TGE (rare in Europe now but still common in some other countries).

Diagnosis

This is based on the occurrence of the diarrhoea post-weaning. Other causes e.g. rotavirus, TGE, PED and salmonella can give similar signs and it is necessary to submit a live or recently dead untreated pig to the laboratory for bacteriological and virological tests to distinguish between them. Determine the antibiotic sensitivity to the *E. coli*.

A simple test to differentiate between virus causes and *E. coli* diarrhoea involves the use of litmus paper to determine whether the scour is an alkaline or an acid consistency. Soak the paper in the scour, *E. coli* diarrhoea is alkaline (blue colour change) whereas viral infections are acid (red colour change).

Treatment

- ❒ Specific treatment will depend on the cause.
- ❒ Sick pigs should be treated individually and group treatment applied to the pigs at risk, ideally by water medication. For example; amoxycillin, apramycin, neomycin, sulphonamides, tiamulin and TMS
- ❒ Add zinc oxide to the weaning ration at a level of 2,500ppm zinc /tonne for 2-3 weeks.
- ❒ If pigs become dehydrated, provide electrolytes in a separate drinker.
- ❒ Suitable antibiotics and medicaments for the treatment of *E. coli* scour (post-weaning).

  Injections:

  Amoxycillin.
  Enrofloxacin.
  Framycetin.
  Gentamycin.
  Tiamulin.
  Trimethoprim/sulpha (TMS).

  In-Feed:

  Amoxycillin 300g/tonne, Apramycin 100g/tonne.
  Combined CTC, penicillin sulphadimidine.
  Furazolidone 400g/tonne.
  Lincomycin 44g / spectinomycin 44g/tonne.
  Neomycin 163g/tonne.
  Tiamulin 100g/tonne.

TMS - variable levels.
Sulphonamides 200-400g/tonne.
Zinc oxide 3.1kg/tonne (Prevention only).

Assess the predisposing factors: *(Refer to Chapter 9 pp285 - 295).*

ELECTROCUTION

This is similar in all pigs see Section 2.

ENCEPHALOMYOCARDITIS (EMC)

This is similar in all pigs see Section 2.

ENZOOTIC PNEUMONIA (EP) - *MYCOPLASMA HYOPNEUMONIAE* INFECTION

Enzootic pneumonia is caused by *Mycoplasma hyopneumoniae.* It is widespread in pig populations and endemic in most herds throughout the world. As an uncomplicated infection in well-housed and well-managed pigs it is relatively unimportant and has only a mild effect on the pig. However if there are other infections present particularly App, Hps, Pasteurella, PRRS or SI, the pneumonia can become more complex with serious effects on the pig.

EP always attacks the lower areas of each lung lobe causing consolidation. The extent of this consolidation in each lobe is scored out of either 5 or 10 depending upon the lobe affected. Thus a severely affected pig with all lobes involved would score 55. This scoring system can be used to assess the severity of disease and its effects on the pig.

If more than 15% of lungs are affected it is highly probable that EP is present in the population. Herds that do not carry *M. hyopneumoniae* rarely show consolidated lesions in more than 1 % and even then they are very small.

If EP is not present in the growing population then the effects of the other respiratory pathogens are greatly reduced. It is therefore considered a primary pathogen that opens up the lung to other infections.

Symptoms

☞ It usually has an incubation period of two to eight weeks before clinical signs are seen but may be longer.

☞ Acute disease is normally only seen in new break-downs of disease.

Over the first six to eight weeks after it enters there may be: (This picture however is extremely variable).

☞ Severe acute pneumonia.

☞ Coughing.

☞ Respiratory distress.

☞ Fever.

☞ High mortality across all ages of stock.

☞ Chronic disease is the normal picture when the organism has been present in the herd for some considerable time.

Maternal antibody is passed via colostrum to the piglets. It disappears from seven to twelve weeks of age after which clinical signs start to appear including:

☞ A prolonged non-productive cough, at least seven to eight coughs per episode, is a common sign around this time, with some pi gs breathing heavily ("thumps").

☞ 30 to 70% of pigs will have lung lesions at slaughter.

Causes / Contributing factors

- It is commonly transmitted through the movement of carrier pigs.
- Wind-borne infection for up to 3km (2 miles) if the climatic conditions are right. The organism dies quickly outside the pig, particularly when dried.
- Incoming pigs.

Increased clinical disease is associated with the following;

- Overcrowding and large group sizes.
- Less than $3m^3$ air space/pig and 0.7m2 floor space/ pig.
- Houses that are too wide for good air flow control.
- Variable temperatures and poor insulation.
- Variable wind speeds and chilling.
- Low temperature, low humidity environments.
- High levels of carbon dioxide and ammonia.
- High dust and bacteria levels in the air.

- Pig movement, stress and mixing.
- Housing with a continuous throughput of pigs.
- Other concurrent diseases particularly PRRS, App, flu, and aujeszky's disease.
- Poor nutrition and dietary changes at susceptible times.

Diagnosis

This is based on the clinical picture and examination of the lungs at post-mortem examination or at slaughter, combined sometimes with histology of the lesions. However, these do not provide a specific diagnosis and in the herds supplying breeding stock or in special cases (e.g. litigation) it may be necessary to confirm the diagnosis by carrying out one or more of the following tests: Serological (ELISA) tests, microscopic examination of stained touch preparations (TPs) of the cut surface of the lungs, fluorescent antibody tests (FATs), polymerase chain reaction (PCRs) tests and finally culture and identification of *Mycoplasma hyopneumoniae*.

These tests are not widely available and many diagnostic laboratories cannot do them. The PCR is probably the most sensitive. FAT, serology and cultures are used in Denmark, but only FATs are available in many laboratories.

EP must be differentiated from flu, PRRS, Hps and other mycoplasma infections. Laboratory tests are required to differentiate them. Furthermore, all or some of these may occur as mixed infections together with *Mycoplasma hyopneumoniae.*

Treatment

May be required if:

There is variable growth in pigs from 10 to 20 weeks of age.

More than 2.5% of the pig population requires individual treatment.

Lung scores more than 15.

In acute break-downs, consider the following:

- ❒ Medicate pigs between weaning and 16 weeks of age for 4 to 8 weeks with 500g/tonne of CTC or OTC and then reduce this to 200-300g/tonne.
- ❒ Inject severely affected individual pigs with either long-acting

OTC, tiamulin, lincomycin or penicillin/streptomycin.

- ❒ If pigs become affected soon after weaning inject with OTC LA at weaning time or one week prior to the onset of disease.

In herds in which EP has become endemic

- ❒ Identify the point at which disease is occurring and apply strategic medication, either in feed, in water or by injection using the drugs outlined above.
- ❒ For strategic medication use tetracyclines 500-800g/tonne, 220g/tonne of lincomycin or 100g/tonne of tiamulin and feed for 7 to 10 days commencing one to three weeks prior to the anticipated time of the disease starting.

Eperythrozoonosis (Epe)

Eperythrozoonosis is caused by a small rickettsial bacterium called *Eperythrozoon suis* (Epe) which attaches itself to the red cells in the blood, damaging them and causing them to break apart. This causes anaemia which may lead to jaundice.

The disease is somewhat of an enigma because the organism is widespread and many healthy pigs examined are shown to be infected. The significance of the organism in relation to disease must be questioned.

Epe can cross the placenta and be responsible for poor pale pigs at birth and high pre-weaning mortality.

Symptoms

The clinical picture varies.

- ☞ In weaners the acute disease is manifest by primary anaemia.
- ☞ In growers it leads to slow growth and poor-doing pigs.
- ☞ The presence of anaemic and possibly slightly yellow-skinned recently weaned pigs.
- ☞ Pale pigs.
- ☞ Slow or variable growth.
- ☞ Ear necrosis.
- ☞ Enteritis.
- ☞ Fever.
- ☞ Pneumonia.

- Poor pigs, wasting, hairy.
- Pot bellied pigs.
- Scour.

Causes / Contributing factors

- Epe suis is spread by inoculation.
- Biting insects.
- Fighting and trauma.

Diagnosis

In trying to arrive at a diagnosis, the following should be considered.

- The clinical picture.
- The identification of the organism in blood smears stained with Wright's stain. Fifty microscopic fields should be exam ined before a negative diagnosis is arrived at.
- Serological tests, including an ELISA, are still unreliable but are being improved.
- Evidence of other causes of anaemia (e.g. iron/copper defi ciency).
- Examination of blood samples for packed cell volume and haemoglobin levels.

Epe has to be distinguished from chronic respiratory disease, glässers disease, leptospirosis, chronic enteritis, pale piglet syndrome (haemorrhages) and porcine enteropathy.

Treatment

Consider the following.

- ❐ Inject piglets with oxytetracycline at 10mg/kg daily for 4 days or use long-acting preparations, three injections each two days apart.
- ❐ In-feed medicate sows at 800gms/tonne of OTC for 4 weeks and repeat again 4 weeks later.
- ❐ Arsanilic acid in-feed at 85gms/tonne is reported to have an effect but in many countries there is no licensed product in food producing animals. Where it is available it is probably the drug of choice.
- ❐ The response to other drugs is poor.

Erysipelas

This is a common disease caused by the bacterium *Erysipelothrix insidiosa*. It is a sub-clinical inhabitant of the tonsils of most healthy swine and is passed out in faeces or via the mouth. The bacterium alone can cause the disease but concurrent virus infections, such as PRRS or influenza, may trigger off outbreaks. The bacteria invade the blood stream through a variety of routes including a break in the skin or via the wall of the digestive tract and a septicaemia develops. The incubation period is 24 to 48 hours.

Symptoms

Acute infection:

☞ Sudden death.

☞ Acutely ill pigs running high temperatures.

☞ Characteristic skin lesions may also be evident as large 10 to 50mm raised diamond shaped areas over the body that may turn from red to black. They may be easier to feel than to see in the early stages and often resolve over 7 - 10 days.

Commonly the disease is less acute and mild.

☞ Skin lesions may appear but the pigs may not appear to be ill in spite of a high temperature 42ºC (107ºF).

☞ The organism may settle in the joints causing chronic arthritis and swellings which can be responsible for condemnations at slaughter.

☞ Lameness.

Causes / Contributing factors

- The movement of pigs involving mixing and stress.
- Sudden changes in temperature and warm summer weather.
- Wet dirty pens.
- Water systems that have become contaminated with the organism.
- Sudden changes in diet.
- Continually populated houses with no all-in, all-out procedures and disinfection.
- Virus infections particularly PRRS and flu.
- Common in straw based systems.

Diagnosis

The typical clinical signs may suggest erysipelas. The skin lesions are diagnostic but for confirmation, tissue samples should be submitted to a laboratory. The organism is easily cultured and identified.

Treatment

- The drug of choice is penicillin which gives a rapid response. If the pig is acutely ill, twice daily injections of short-acting penicillin should be used initially. Continue antibiotic cover for four days. If the pig is less acutely ill long acting penicillin can be used. Clinically the pig returns to normal in 24 hours.
- Where large numbers of pigs are involved it may be necessary to inject all the pigs in the groups at risk.
- Treatment can be started in the drinking water and can be continued in the feed. Phenoxymethyl penicillin (Pen V) at 200g/tonne or tetracyclines at 500g/tonne should be effective. Pen. V can also be used for prevention in the face of an outbreak.
- In individual outbreaks finishing pens should be washed and disinfected between batches.
- In continual outbreaks in growing pigs it may be necessary to vaccinate pigs at 8 weeks and possibly again at 10-12 weeks of age. Normally, pigs are not vaccinated before 8 weeks because colostrum antibodies reduce the vaccine response.

Fever

This is similar in all pigs see Section 2.

Foot-and-Mouth Disease (FMD)

(See Chapter 12 pp406)

This disease should always be considered if sudden widespread lameness appears with vesicles or blisters on the snout, tongue and tops of the claws. In most countries it is notifiable and if suspected must be reported to the authorities immediately. Salivation is an obvious symptom.

FRACTURES

(Chapter 9 pp 313)

Fractures are common in growing pigs due to environmental trauma and where appropriate high stocking densities.

Symptoms

- ☞ The onset of clinical signs is invariably sudden.
- ☞ The animal is unable to rise on its own without difficulty.
- ☞ A significant feature is the reluctance to place any weight on the affected leg and lameness.
- ☞ The muscles and tissues over the fracture site are often swollen and painful.
- ☞ The pig is very reluctant to move unless on three legs.
- ☞ Crepitus or the rubbing together of the two broken ends of the bone can often be felt.
- ☞ The pig adopts a dog sitting position.
- ☞ In chronic cases joints may be swollen and abscessed.

Causes / Contributing factors

- Trauma.
- Fighting.
- Bone disease i.e. osteomalacia.
- Calcium phosphorus and vitamin D deficiency.
- Leg weakness - Osteochondrosis (OCD).

Diagnosis

This is based upon the history, symptoms and palpation to detect crepitus. Fractures must be differentiated from acute laminitis, arthritis, and muscle tearing.

Treatment

- ❐ Animals with fractures should be slaughtered/destroyed on the farm.

FROSTBITE

This is similar in all pigs see Section 2.

FUNGAL POISONING - MYCOTOXICOSIS

This is similar in all pigs see Section 2.

Gastric Ulcers

(Chapter 9 pp 314)

Erosion and ulceration of the lining of the stomach is a common condition in growing pigs. It occurs in the area where the oesophagus enters the stomach. In the early stages the area becomes roughened and gradually changes as the surface becomes eroded until it is actively ulcerated. Intermittent haemorrhage may then take place leading to anaemia, or massive haemorrhage may occur resulting in death. The incidence at slaughter in growing pigs is up to 60%.

Symptoms

Acute form:

☞ Previously healthy animals are found dead.

☞ The most striking sign is the paleness of the carcass due to internal haemorrhage.

Less acute form:

☞ The affected pig is pale.

☞ Weak.

☞ Shows breathlessness.

☞ Grinding of the teeth.

☞ Vomiting.

☞ The passing of dark faeces containing digested blood is often a persistent symptom.

☞ Usually the temperature is normal.

In chronic cases:

☞ The pig has an intermittent appetite and may lose weight.

Causes / Contributing factors

These may be nutritional and related to the physical properties of the feed, managemental, or triggered by other diseases.

- Nutritional factors include:
  - Low protein diets.
  - Low fibre diets. (Introduction of straw reduces the incidence).
  - High energy diets.
  - High levels of wheat in excess of 55%.
  - Deficiencies of vitamin E or selenium.
  - Diets containing high levels of iron, copper or calcium.

  - Diets low in zinc.
  - Diets with high levels of unsaturated fats.
  - Diets based on whey and skimmed milk.
- Physical aspects of the feed.
  - Size of feed particle - the more finely ground the meal the smaller the particle size and the higher the incidence of ulcers. This is still the case if the finely ground feed is then pelleted.
  - Rolling cereals as distinct from grinding them will often pro duce a dramatic drop in the incidence but the penalties of feed use have to be taken into consideration.
  - Pelleting feeds in itself increases the incidence. Feed meal.
  - However, sometimes changing from pellets to meal itself causes problems. A compromise is to feed alternatively.
- Managemental factors that increase the incidence:
  - Irregular feeding patterns and shortage of feeder space.
  - Periods of starvation or lack of water.
  - Increased stocking densities and movement of pigs or any other undue stresses including poor stockmanship.
  - Transportation.
- Other diseases.
  - There is a clear relationship between outbreaks of pneumo nia and the incidence of gastric ulceration.
  - Ulceration may occur following bacterial septicaemias such as those associated with erysipelas and swine fever.

Diagnosis

This is based on the clinical signs and post mortem lesions. A sample of faeces should be examined for the presence of blood and to eliminate parasites. An examination of stomachs at slaughter should be carried out.

Gastric ulcers must be differentiated from haemorrhage of the bowel, eperythrozoonosis, the red stomach worm *Hyostrongylus rubidus*, chronic mange and porcine enteropathy.

Treatment

❒ Move the affected animal from its existing housing into a loose

bedded peaceful environment. Correct predisposing factors.
- Feed a weaner type diet containing highly digestible materials.
- Inject multi vitamins and in particular vitamin E together with 0.5 to 1g of iron intramuscularly and repeat on a weekly basis.
- Add an extra 100g vitamin E / tonne to the diet for two months and assess the results.
- Cull severely affected pigs.

Glässers Disease (*Haemophilus Parasuis* Hps)

(Chapter 9 pp 315)

This is caused by the bacterium *Haemophilus parasuis.* It is ubiquitous, found throughout the world and is present even in high health herds. If such herds are set up using SPF or MEW techniques and are free from Hps it can be devastating when they first become contaminated.

In the majority of herds in which the bacterium is endemic, sows produce a strong maternal immunity which normally persists in their offspring until 8 to 12 weeks of age preventing disease. Disease may however be seen in sucking pigs. Pigs usually become sub-clinically infected when still protected by maternal antibody. If however the maternal immunity wears off before they become infected they may develop severe disease. This is usually sometime after weaning. It can also become a secondary organism particularly in enzootic pneumonia.

Symptoms

- Pigs with glässers disease become rapidly depressed or may be just found dead.
- Elevated temperature.
- Stop eating.
- Reluctant to rise.
- Fever.
- Nervous signs including meningitis.
- Poor pigs, wasting, hairy often result.

In young growing pigs the following are common:

- Fever.

- ☞ Mild meningitis.
- ☞ Arthritis.
- ☞ Lameness.
- ☞ Pneumonia.
- ☞ Heart sac infection.
- ☞ Peritonitis and pleurisy.
- ☞ A characteristic feature is a short cough of only 2-3 episodes.

Causes

- It is respiratory spread. Disease may be precipitated by PRRS, flu or EP.
- Poor environments, draughts etc. predispose.
- Stress.

Diagnosis

This is based on clinical observations, post-mortem examinations and isolation of the organism in the laboratory.

Glässers disease must be distinguished from *Actinobacillus suis*. infection, mulberry heart disease, streptococcal meningitis and bacterial septicaemias.

Treatment

- ❒ Hps has a wide antibiotic sensitivity including amoxycillin, ampicillin, OTC, sulphonamides, penicillin and ceftiofur.
- ❒ Treatment is best by injection and must be given early.
- ❒ Treat for 2 to 3 days.
- ❒ Medicate the water with amoxycillin or phenoxymethyl penicillin for 4-5 days over the period of risk.

Greasy Pig Disease - Exudative Epidermitis

(Chapter 9 pp 316)

This is caused by the bacterium *Staphylococcus hyicus* which invades abraded skin. It is a normal inhabitant of the skin. The *Staphylococcus* produces toxins which are absorbed into the system and damage the liver and kidneys.

Symptoms

- ☞ Usually commence about 3 days after weaning with localised, brown areas of infection around the face or on the legs, where the skin has been damaged.

- The skin along the flanks the belly and between the legs changes to a brown colour gradually involving the whole of the body.
- The skin becomes wrinkled with flaking of large areas.
- It progresses to a dark greasy texture and in severe cases turns black.
- Such cases usually die due to the toxins produce by the staphylococci organisms.
- In nurseries up to 15% of the population may be involved.
- Dehydration is common.

Causes / Contributing factors

- Abrasions arising from poor concrete surfaces or rough metal floors.
- Mange giving rise to skin damage.
- Damage to the face by metal feeding troughs can precipitate disease.
- Abnormal behaviour - tail biting, ear biting, navel sucking, flank biting.
- Badly clipped teeth at birth.

Diagnosis

This is based on the characteristic skin lesions. *(See Chapter 10 pp 356).* In an outbreak it is helpful to culture the organism and carry out an antibiotic sensitivity test. A moist wet area should be identified, the overlying scab removed and a swab rubbed well into the infected area. This should be sent to the laboratory in transport medium for culture and antibiotic sensitivity tests.

Treatment

- Inject affected piglets daily for 5 days, or on alternate days with a long-acting antibiotic to which the organism is sensitive.
- Antibiotics include; amoxycillin, OTC, ceftiofur, cephalexin, gentamycin, lincomycin or penicillin.
- Topical application can also be of use. Novobiocin can be mixed with mineral oil and sprayed onto the skin or the piglets dipped into a solution of it.
- Pigs become dehydrated and should be offered electrolytes by mouth.

HAEMATOMA

(Chapter 9 pp 317)

A haematoma is a pocket of blood beneath the skin. It is often seen in the growing period and the most common site is the ear.

Symptoms

☞ Large swellings which develop suddenly.

☞ The swellings contain blood or serum.

Causes / Contributing factors

- Fighting.
- Trauma.

Diagnosis

Clinical signs. Differentiate from an abscess, test with a needle and syringe.

Treatment

❒ In most cases these will resolve over two to three weeks once the blood has formed a clot and the serum is absorbed. The clot is then slowly removed.

❒ Large haematomas on the ears cause considerable discomfort and in such cases the pig should be suitably restrained and a needle entered into the swelling. The removed fluid shows if the blood has clotted.

❒ In the growing pig it may be advisable to lance the ear at the tip leaving a 20mm open incision to allow drainage.

LAMENESS

(Chapter 9 pp 317)

This is prevalent in growing pigs with levels ranging from 1 to 5%. If more than 2% of pigs are recorded lame per month further investigations are necessary.

Lameness can account for significant losses in growing pigs either because the pigs are unfit to travel on welfare grounds and require to be destroyed, or they are part or totally condemned at slaughter. Early identification of lame animals and their removal to hospital pens for treatment is a vital part of the control and healing process.

Symptoms

- ☞ Pig may be off food.
- ☞ Sometimes fever.
- ☞ Reluctance to stand. Difficulty moving.
- ☞ Swollen joints.
- ☞ Evidence of other diseases.

Causes / Contributing factors

- Arthritis caused by bacteria. *
- Back muscle necrosis - a stress related disease.
- Bursitis. *
- Bush foot. *
- Erysipelas. *
- Foot-and-mouth disease and swine vesicular disease in those countries where they occur.
- Fractures. *
- Glässers disease.
- High stocking densities.
- Leg weakness or Osteochondrosis. *
- Mycoplasma arthritis. *
- Nutritional deficiencies.
- Porcine stress syndrome associated with the halothane gene.
- Split horn.
- Tail biting (see vice - abnormal behaviour).
- Torn ligaments or muscles.
- Trauma. * (Stocking density and mixing are the two major factors that precipitate traumatic disease).
- Poor floor surfaces.
- Fighting.
- Cuts or breaks in the skin related to sharp projections.

Diagnosis

This is based on the clinical signs.

Treatment

- ❒ Specific treatment will depend on the cause.
- ❒ Assess response to penicillin and lincomycin.
- ❒ Move pigs to hospital pen.

Leg Weakness - Osteochondrosis (OCD)

(Chapter 7 pp 211)

Leg deformities are common in the rapidly growing pig but are usually of no commercial consequence. Separation of the head of the femur at the growth plate however occurs in rapidly growing pigs on some farms.

Symptoms

- ☞ Acute cases are characterised by the sudden onset of acute lameness, highlighted by poor conformation of legs, bending of bones and dropped pasterns.
- ☞ The pig refuses to put the foot to the floor.
- ☞ Fractures in the hip, knee and shoulder joints. Evident at slaughter or post mortem.
- ☞ Long-term the joint changes may lead to arthritis.

Causes / Contributing factors

- ◆ High stocking density.
- ◆ Environmental factors that cause the foot to slip on the floor.
- ◆ Rapid weight gain.

Diagnosis

This is by the clinical signs.

Treatment

- ❒ In early cases move pigs to well bedded straw pens.
- ❒ If fractures destroy.

Leptospirosis

(Chapter 6 pp186)

Growing pigs are occasionally exposed to *Leptospira ictero-haemorrhagiae* from the urine of rats.

Remember that this disease can be transmitted to people.

Symptoms

- ☞ Acute jaundice.
- ☞ Haemorrhage.
- ☞ Rapid death.
- ☞ Pale pigs.

Causes / Contributing factors

- Rats, mice and dogs can be reservoirs of infection.
- Poor floor surfaces allow urine to pool.
- Spread in urine.

Diagnosis

This is by clinical signs. Laboratory tests are required.

Treatment

❒ Antibiotics amoxycillin and oxytetracycline are effective.

LYMPHOSARCOMA

This is a tumour affecting all the lymph glands throughout the body but particularly those of the intestines and lungs. The condition is very occasionally seen in the Large White where a hereditary component is thought to be involved.

Reported levels of lymphosarcoma found at slaughter are extremely low (0.002%).

Symptoms

☞ These are usually seen in young growing pigs.
☞ Pale skin.
☞ Sometimes slightly jaundiced.
☞ Loss of weight.
☞ Pot bellied appearance.
☞ Enlarged glands may be seen in the neck.
☞ Most pigs die within 4-5 months.

Causes / Contributing factors

- Unknown but thought to be associated with a virus and genetic predisposition.

Diagnosis

This is based on clinical tests confirmed by post mortem examinations.

Treatment

❒ None. Destroy affected pigs.

Mange Mites (Sarcoptes Scabiei)

(Chapter 11 pp385)

This is caused by the tiny mite *Sarcoptes scabiei* which burrows into the skin. See also Section 2.

Symptoms

- ☞ Its presence affects food conversion and daily gain, particularly if the weight of infection is heavy.
- ☞ Tiny red pimples over the skin.
- ☞ Irritation and rubbing/scratching.
- ☞ Ear shaking.
- ☞ Chronic condition - Thick asbestos like scabs, mainly on the ears, often with slight bleeding and constant rubbing.

Causes / Contributing factors

- Disease only present if the mite exists in the herd.
- If routine control and treatment is not carried out severe disease results.

Diagnosis

Clinical signs and skin changes indicate the presence of the mite. Skin scrapings should be submitted to the laboratory for microscopic examination.

Treatment

- ❒ Topical with amitraz or diazinon.
- ❒ Injections using ivermectins.
- ❒ In-feed using ivermectins.

Mastitis

This is similar in all pigs see Section 2.

Meningitis

See **streptococcal infections** and Section 2 (meningitis)

Middle Ear Infections

(Chapter 9 pp 319)

This is caused by a variety of bacteria, that gain access to the middle part of the ear which is responsible for balance. Infection probably arises from the tonsils at the back of the throat and travels down the eustachian tube to the middle part of the ear. The condition is sporadic but common particularly in weaners. If treatment is prompt there is usually a good response. If treatment is delayed there is the risk that infection will spread from the middle ear into the inner ear and inwards to cause meningitis

Symptoms

- ☞ The pig stands with its head to one side often shaking.
- ☞ As the disease progresses there is a gradual loss of co-ordination until ultimately the pig walks around in a circle eventually falling over.
- ☞ Nervous signs i.e. meningitis may result

Causes / Contributing factors

Disease may result from:

- Mange.
- Skin trauma.
- Vice - Abnormal behaviour.
- Fighting.
- Greasy pig disease.
- Joint infections.
- PRRS infection.

Diagnosis

Clinical signs. Bacteriological examinations should be carried out if many pigs are involved.

Treatment

- ❒ In acute cases it is necessary to inject the pig twice daily for the first two days with penicillin/streptomycin or amoxycillin and then follow up with long-acting injections. Long acting OTC can also be used.
- ❒ Treatment must continue for 7-10 days and complete recovery may take up to 3 weeks.
- ❒ Consider preventative medication using amoxycillin long-acting injections given strategically just prior to disease onset.

Mortality

(Chapter 9 pp 319)

Excessive mortality is a significant economic loss and if the levels in the herd are above an acceptable target (3 - 6%) then the reasons for the excess should be identified. For each pig that is found dead or destroyed note the date, age and weight, the house in which it died, the believed cause of death and any comments. Such a system can easily be recorded on cards. The quality of nursing care given to sick pigs can significantly affect the target levels at the upper limit. The movement to and reasons for sick pigs entering hospital pens should also be recorded.

Recorded causes of death.

(i.e. those that may be readily diagnosed by an experienced pig person).

The Weaner

Acute enteritis.
Fighting.
Glässers disease.
Meningitis.
Miscellaneous causes.
Oedema disease.
Post-weaning diarrhoea.
Rectal prolapse.
Stress.
Respiratory disease.
Vice (abnormal behaviour).
Welfare culls (culled on welfare grounds).
Unknown.

The Grower Pig

Abscess.
Bloody diarrhoea.
Enteric problems.
Erysipelas.
Fighting.
Gastric ulcers.
Miscellaneous causes.
Pale pig.
Rectal prolapse.
Rectal stricture.
Respiratory disease.
Salt poisoning/water depri vation.
Stress/torsion of the stomach and intestines.
Vice (abnormal behaviour).
Welfare culls (culled on welfare grounds).
Unknown.

Mulberry Heart Disease (Vitamin E / Selenium Deficiency)

(Chapter 9 pp 320)

Vitamin E is widespread in feed stuffs including vegetable oils, cereals and green plants but problems arise often from using polyunsaturated fats in diets as sources of energy which destroys the vitamins. Vitamin E is necessary for the optimum function and metabolism of the nervous, muscular, circulatory and immune systems. It helps to maintain the integral structure of muscles in the digestive and reproductive systems and is involved in the synthesis of certain amino acids and vitamin C. It has a close relationship with selenium metabolism. The less selenium in the diet the greater is the requirement for vitamin E.

The recommended requirements are 100iu/kg in the grower ration and 60iu/kg in the finisher ration. These levels are probably higher than those necessary for maximum growth, which may be 50% less. When polyunsaturated fatty acids (PUFA) are added to diets 3iu of vitamin E should be added for each g of PUFA.

Symptoms

Clinical signs and post mortem lesions vary according to the system affected and include:

- Sudden death in rapid growing pigs without any prior clinical signs.
- Increased levels of concurrent diseases.
- Gastric ulcers.
- Pale pigs.

Post-mortem symptoms are characteristic and include:

- Large amounts of fluid around the heart and lungs.
- Haemorrhagic and pale areas in heart muscle.
- Fluid in the abdomen with pieces of fibrin.
- Pale muscle areas (necrosis) particularly in the lumber muscles and hind muscles of the leg which contain excesses amounts of fluid.
- If the liver is involved it is enlarged and mottled with areas of haemorrhage interspersed with pale areas.

Vitamin E and selenium related diseases

- Gastric ulcers - These are often caused by stress but the incidence increases where vitamin E levels are low.
- Hepatosis dietetica - Death of liver cells.
- Muscular or nutritional dystrophy. Degeneration of skeletal, smooth or cardiac muscle fibres. Fluid often accumulates around muscles.
- Mulberry heart disease (MHD). A disease of the heart muscle resulting in sudden death.

Causes / Contributing factors

- Diet i.e. high levels of fat.
- Vitamin A deficiency.
- Vitamin E and selenium deficiency.
- Rapid growth may be a contributing factor.
- High stocking densities may predispose.
- Grains stored with high moisture content in high temperatures and with fungal growth may have low levels of vitamin E.

Diagnosis

Accurate diagnosis requires histological examinations of the liver, heart or skeletal muscle. Serum samples should be taken from pigs at risk and tested for levels of vitamin E.

Treatment

- ❒ Where a population is at risk inject all the pigs with vitamin E/selenium e.g. dystocel, 70iu vitamin E and 1.5mg per 50kg is adequate, but seek veterinary advice.
- ❒ Water soluble preparations are sometimes available as alternatives.
- ❒ Multi-vitamins that include vitamin E and or selenium may be used. Refer to the recommended treatment levels on the bottle label.
- ❒ Move individual pigs to hospital pens for treatment.
- ❒ Increase vitamin E levels growing rations by 100-150iu/kg.

Muscle Tearing

This is similar in all pigs see Section 2.

Mycoplasma Arthritis (*Mycoplasma Hyosynoviae* Infection)

(Chapter 9 pp 321)

Mycoplasma hyosynoviae is ubiquitous and most, if not all herds are infected with it. It is a respiratory spread disease, the organism being found in the upper respiratory tract nose and tonsils, although the damage is to joints and tendon sheaths rather than the respiratory system itself.

It may be present in some herds and cause no clinical signs and yet in others cause severe disease. Infection with or without disease takes place in the growing pig from approximately 8 to 30 weeks of age.

Symptoms

- Reluctance to rise.
- Trembling.
- Considerable amount of pain particularly when standing.
- Only stand for short periods of time.
- Temperature normal or slightly elevated.
- Lameness swollen joints.

Causes / Contributing factors

- The quality of housing - in particular low temperatures and draughts may act as trigger factors.
- Mixing and fighting causing stress.
- High stocking densities.
- Poor ventilation.
- Sudden nutritional changes.

Diagnosis

This is based on lameness and the response to either lincomycin or tiamulin therapy. Joint fluid can be aspirated and examined for antibodies and isolation of the organism. Serology is not much help because sub-clinical infection is common and so healthy animals often have antibody titres but rising titres in blood samples taken two weeks apart together with typical symptoms strongly suggest disease. In problem herds post-mortem examinations may be required to differentiate from other diseases.

Mycoplasma hyosynoviae arthritis must be differentiated from muscle damage, leg weakness, trauma, erysipelas and glässers disease.

Treatment

- ❒ Give lincomycin or tiamulin injections daily for 4 days. There should be a good response within 24 to 36 hours.
- ❒ Treatment is most effective if given early.
- ❒ Give in feed medication strategically commencing 7 days before the expected disease outbreak and continue for 14 days using 220g/tonne of lincomycin or 500-800g/tonne of OTC or CTC.
- ❒ An alternate strategy is to medicate the ration at half these levels and feed for 5-7 weeks.
- ❒ Remember that this is a respiratory spread disease and other control factors need to be considered.

Oedema Disease (OD) - Bowel Oedema (EDEMA)

(Chapter 9 pp 322)

This is also called gut oedema. It is caused by certain serotypes of *E. coli* bacteria that produce a powerful toxin. These toxins damage the walls of small blood vessels including those in the brain and cause fluid or oedema to accumulate in the tissues of the stomach and the large bowel. Damage to the blood vessels in the brain results in characteristic nervous signs. Disease is now uncommon and generally only seen 1 to 4 weeks after weaning, the peak being at 14 days.

Symptoms

- ☞ Sometimes the only sign is a good pig found dead.

Typical live affected pigs show:

- ☞ A staggering gate.
- ☞ Puffy eyelids giving a sleepy appearance.
- ☞ An abnormal high pitched squeak.
- ☞ Pigs stop eating.
- ☞ In the later stages become partially paralysed and go off their legs.
- ☞ Sometimes with nervous symptoms. Muscle twitching, fits.

- Diarrhoea is not a feature.
- Breathing difficulties become evident.
- The damage to the brain is irreversible and most pigs die.
- Lameness.

Causes / Contributing factors

- Associated with weaning and changes of diet.

Diagnosis

This is made from the typical clinical signs, the sudden appearance of disease after weaning, post-mortem examinations showing oedema (fluid in tissues) of the greater curvature of the stomach wall, coiled colon and eyelids and isolation of the haemolytic *E. coli* serotypes from the anterior small intestine.

Treatment

By the time the clinical signs are seen it is too late and most pigs die. Treatment routines are aimed at preventing the organism establishing itself and also reducing the weight of infection. The general principles of controlling coliform infections and post-weaning diarrhoea should be followed.

- Isolate the organism and determine the antibiotic sensitivity.
- Identify the stage (e.g. 10 days post-weaning) when disease first appears and apply either in-feed or water medication 3 to 5 days before this.
- In-feed antibiotics of value include apramycin 100g/tonne, framycetin 100g/tonne, neomycin 163g/tonne. Alternatively apramycin, neomycin or trimethoprim/sulpha can be used in the water.

The disease is most difficult to deal with and often preventative medication and treatment are unsuccessful.

Osteomalacia (OM)

This is similar in all pigs see Section 2.

Parasites (Internal)

(Chapter 11)

Internal parasites are an uncommon problem in the weaned,

growing and finisher pig unless they are housed in continuously occupied straw based or bare concrete pens. *Chapter 11* details parasites in depth.

Symptoms

☞ Coccidiosis could cause diarrhoea within 7 to 10 days of entry to continually used pens.

☞ Strongyle infections (poor growth and sloppy faeces) within 3 to 4 weeks

☞ Coughing.

☞ Blood in faeces.

☞ Pneumonia / Heavy breathing.

☞ Pale pigs.

Causes / Contributing factors

- Continuously used pens predispose.
- Wet dirty floors.
- Carrier pigs.

Diagnosis

Laboratory examination of faeces for worm eggs.

Treatment

❒ Identify the specific parasite. Most worms respond to anthelmintics by injection or in-feed such as bendazoles or ivermectins.

❒ Adopt all-in, all-out procedures to break the cycle.

PASTEURELLOSIS

(Chapter 9 pp 323)

Non-toxin-producing strains of *Pasteurella multocidia* bacteria are commonly involved in respiratory disease in pigs. They can cause pneumonia in their own right but are usually secondary opportunist invaders associated with primary EP or PRRS infections. The condition usually affects pigs between 10 and 18 weeks of age.

Symptoms

Acute disease is characterised by:

☞ Severe sudden pneumonia affecting all the lung tissue.

- High temperatures.
- Discharges from the nose.
- High mortality.
- Pigs show rapid breathing.
- Discoloured skin particularly on the extremities of the ears (caused by toxins or heart sac infections).

Sub acute disease is characterised by:

- Pneumonia which is less severe but often complicated by heart sac inflammation and pleurisy.
- Coughing.
- Discharges from the nose.
- Emaciation.
- Increased mortality.

Causes / Contributing factors

- Concurrent disease such as PRRS, Flu and EP predispose.

Diagnosis

This is carried out by post-mortem examination and isolation of the organism from the lungs.

Treatment

- ❒ Because the organism is usually secondary to EP, antibiotic treatments should be those used for EP.
- ❒ Inject individual pigs daily with oxytetracycline, penicillin, dimycin. Antibiotic sensitivities are usually wide.
- ❒ In-feed medicate with antibiotics or by water in acute outbreaks.

Peritonitis

This is similar in all pigs see Section 2.

Pneumonia (Chronic Respiratory Disease)

(Chapter 9 pp328)

Of all the diseases that affect growing and finishing pigs, chronic respiratory disease is the most economically important. It is extremely common and can be difficult to prevent and control.

Growth rates and feed-intake are depressed together with poor feed efficiency and in some herds there is heavy mortality. The control of respiratory disease requires an understanding of the complexities and interaction between the organisms that are present, the pig and the management of the environment.

Pneumonia is affected by;

- The presence of respiratory pathogenic organisms.
- The virulence of the pathogens present.
- The level of the pathogens in the house environment.
- The immunity of the pig and the time of exposure to the organisms
- The presence of secondary opportunistic bacteria.
- The interactions between management, environment, the diseases and the pig.

Symptoms

☞ Coughing.
☞ Rapid breathing.
☞ Dehydration.
☞ Inappetence.
☞ Discharges from the eyes.
☞ Poor circulation.
☞ Blue discoloration.
☞ Loss of condition.
☞ Huddling.

Causes / Contributing factors

- Diseases are commonly transmitted through the movement of carrier pigs.
- Incoming pigs.

Increased clinical disease is associated with the following;

- Overcrowding and large group sizes.
- Less than $3m^3$ air space/pig and $0.7m^2$ floor space/ pig.
- Houses that are too wide for good air flow control.
- Variable temperatures and poor insulation.
- Variable wind speeds and chilling.
- Low temperature, low humidity environments.
- High levels of carbon dioxide and ammonia.

- High dust and bacteria levels in the air.
- Pig movement, stress and mixing.
- Housing with a continuous throughput of pigs.
- A combination of diseases, particularly PRRS, App, flu, and aujeszky's.
- Poor nutrition and dietary changes at susceptible times.

Diagnosis

To differentiate causes laboratory examinations are necessary.

Treatment

- ❒ Identify the bacteria and medicate with antibiotics.
- ❒ Common ones used include CTC, OTC, tiamulin, lincomycin, trimethoprim/sulpha, penicillin/dimycin.
- ❒ Treat individual sick pigs by injection for 3 - 4 days. This is the most effective and cost effective method.
- ❒ Water medicate in acute outbreaks.
- ❒ In feed medicate for periods of 2 -4 weeks or strategically medicate.
- ❒ Provide good nursing. Hospitalise ill pigs.
- ❒ Provide easy access to food and water.

Porcine Cytomegalovirus (PCMV)

This is similar in all pigs see Section 2.

Porcine Enteropathy (PE)

(Chapter 9 pp 324)

This comprises a group of conditions involving pathological changes in the small intestine associated with the bacterium *Lawsonia intracellularis*. This exists on most if not all farms. Disease takes four different forms: porcine intestinal adenopathy (PIA) an abnormal proliferation of the cells that line the intestines; necrotic enteritis (NE) where the proliferated cells of the small intestine die and slough off with a gross thickening of the small intestine (hosepipe gut); regional ileitis (RI), inflammation of the terminal part of the small intestine and proliferative haemorrhagic enteropathy (PHE). In the latter there is massive bleeding into the small intestine, hence the common name bloody gut and is the commonest form in growing pigs. The other three forms are rarer and progress from PIA. PHE is more common in 60-90kg pigs and gilts.

The organism is impossible to keep out of farms probably because it also infects other species. Infected faeces are the major vehicle for spread around the farm.

Symptoms

Clinical signs of PIA, NE, RI are different from PHE.

PIA:

- ☞ The pig appears clinically normal.
- ☞ Initially eats well.
- ☞ Chronic diarrhoea.
- ☞ Gradual wasting.
- ☞ Loss of condition.
- ☞ In some cases a pot bellied appearance.
- ☞ Pigs with the chronic form of the PIA recover over a period of four to six weeks, however there can be considerable losses in feed efficiency and daily gain of up to 0.3 and 80g/day respectively. As a consequence there can be marked variations in sizes of pigs.
- ☞ NI or RI follow from it with similar signs.

PHE is an acute disease:

- ☞ Bloody scour.
- ☞ The pig may die suddenly.
- ☞ Appears very pale and passes black bloody faeces.

Causes / Contributing factors

- Carry over of infection between batches appears to be a main means of spread.
- Associated with continual population of finishing pens.

Diagnosis

This is based on the clinical picture, post-mortem examinations, histology of the gut wall and demonstrating the organism in faeces by an ELISA test. A serological test is also available. Only a few laboratories can do these tests. Tissue cultures have been recently developed.

Treatment

- ❒ The following antibiotics have been shown to be effective. Penicillin, enrofloxacin, erythromycin and chlortetracyline, tiamulin and tilmycosin.
- ❒ Treat individual pigs with injections of long-acting oxytetracycline or penicillin and give 300-800mg of iron dextran.
- ❒ In acute outbreaks medicate the water for 2 to 3 days with OTC or CTC followed by in-feed medication.
- ❒ Virginiamycin - used as a growth promoter could be used to prevent disease.
- ❒ Consider adopting all-in, all-out. procedures.

PORCINE EPIDEMIC DIARRHOEA (PED)

(Chapter 12 - pp 410)

PED is a rapid spreading virus infection of the small intestine. See also Section 2.

Symptoms

- ☞ Acute watery diarrhoea with no blood or mucus.
- ☞ Mortality is usually low but morbidity can be high.
- ☞ When the virus is first introduced on to the farm there is a rapid spread of diarrhoea across all breeding and growing pigs with almost 100% morbidity (pigs affected) within 5 to 10 days. The incubation period is 2 to 4 days.
- ☞ Vomiting.

Causes / Contributing factors

- Disease may be perpetuated as susceptible pigs enter the finishing herd.
- Disease normally only seen when virus first enters the herd.

Diagnosis

This is based on the history, clinical signs and examination of faeces samples for evidence of porcine epidemic diarrhoea virus by ELISA tests or electron microscopy. Post-mortem examination of dead pigs and laboratory tests on the small intestine may be necessary to confirm the diagnosis.

PED must be differentiated from TGE by laboratory tests.

Treatment

- ❒ The growing pig normally recovers without treatment unless concurrent infections such as swine dysentery are present. In such cases antibiotics in the water or preventative medication in-feed maybe required.
- ❒ All-in, all-out procedures with disinfection will often break the cycle. The virus is easily killed by phenolic, chlorine or iodine based disinfectants.

Porcine Reproductive and Respiratory Syndrome (PRRS)

(Chapter 9 pp325)

PRRS (Blue ear disease) is caused by a recently identified arterivirus.

This virus has a particular affinity for macrophages cells particularly those found in the lung. Macrophages are part of the body defences. They ingest and remove invading bacteria and viruses. Those present in the lung are called alveolar macrophages. In contrast to most other bacteria and viruses, macrophages do not destroy the PRRS virus. Instead, the virus multiplies inside them producing more virus in the process the cells die.

Up to 40% of the macrophages are destroyed which removes a major part of the bodies defence mechanism and allows bacteria and other viruses to proliferate and do damage.

A common example of this is the noticeable increase in severity of enzootic pneumonia in grower/finisher units when they become infected with PRRS virus.

PRRS infects all types of herd including high or ordinary health status and both indoor and outdoor units, irrespective of size.

Symptoms

When first introduced into an EP and App free growing herd there may be few signs:

- ☞ A period of slight inappetence.
- ☞ Mild coughing.
- ☞ In some herds there are no symptoms.

If EP and/or virulent App are present but under control in the herd:

- ☞ An acute extensive consolidating pneumonia.
- ☞ Formation of multiple abscesses.
- ☞ Disease becomes evident within 1-3 weeks of weaning.
- ☞ Pigs lose condition.
- ☞ Diarrhoea may be seen.
- ☞ Pale skin.
- ☞ Mild coughing.
- ☞ Sneezing.
- ☞ Discharges from the eyes.
- ☞ Increased respiratory rates.
- ☞ Mortality during this period may reach 12-15%.

Once the acute period of disease has passed through PRRS virus normally only becomes of significance in the early growing period:

- ☞ Severe pneumonia.
- ☞ Periods of inappetence.
- ☞ Wasting.

Pigs become infected as maternal antibody disappears and then remain viraemic for 3 to 4 weeks continually excreting virus.

Clinical disease is seen in pigs 4 to 12 weeks of age:

- ☞ Inappetence.
- ☞ Malabsorption.
- ☞ Wasting.
- ☞ Coughing.
- ☞ Pneumonia.
- ☞ In this post-weaning period mortality can rise up to 12% or more and persist inspite of antibiotic treatments.

Secondary bacterial infections become evident in pigs at a later stage from 12 to 16 weeks of age:

- ☞ Abscesses develop in the lungs and may spread throughout the body.
- ☞ Lameness with abscesses.
- ☞ Poor stunted growth.

Causes / Contributing factors

The following are common methods of spread and contribute to overall disease levels.

- Droplet contamination from older pigs to younger pigs.
- Nasal secretions, saliva, faeces and urine
- Permanently populated houses maintain the virus at high levels, particularly in the first and second stage nurseries.
- Movement of carrier pigs.
- Airborne transmission up to 3km (2 miles).
- Mechanical means via faeces, dust, droplets and contaminated equipment.
- Contaminated boots and clothing.
- Vehicles especially in cold weather.
- Artificial insemination but only if the boar is viraemic. This period is probably only 3-4 days.
- Adult animals excrete virus for much shorter periods of time (14 days) compared to growing pigs which can excrete for 1-2 months.
- The mallard duck and probably other species of bird.

Diagnosis

This is based on the clinical signs, post mortem examinations and the known presence of the virus in the herd or by serological examinations and isolation of the virus in a laboratory.

Treatment

- ❒ In the acute disease when PRRS first enters the farm it is important to cover the period at risk, which is usually six to eight weeks, with in-feed antibiotics or by individual injections and water medication.
- ❒ The broad spectrum antibiotics, tetracyclines, trimethoprim/sulpha, or synthetic penicillins are the drugs of choice for the secondary bacteria (antibiotics have no effect against the virus) but if EP alone is involved tiamulin or lincomycin may be used. If App is active ceftiofur could be a drug of choice for individual treatments. Response to treatment may be slow and poor.
- ❒ In endemic disease preventive medication over the period at risk using 500 to 800g of tetracycline or trimethoprim/sulpha

400g/tonne in-feed may be used but it would be advisable to identify the major bacteria involved and determine their antibiotic sensitivities.

(See also Respiratory disease and control strategies in *Chapter 9 pp 328*).

(Refer to *Chapter 3 pp 94* Segregated Weaning and Disease Control).

Porcine Respiratory Coronavirus (PRCV)

(Chapter 12 pp 411)

PRCV first appeared in pigs some ten years or more ago in Europe. It is related to but distinct from TGE virus, which is another coronavirus. It has been suggested that the virus may have an effect on lung tissue when other respiratory pathogens are present in chronic respiratory disease complexes.

Symptoms

- Herds exposed for the first time have few if any signs of disease.
- A transient coughing lasting only a few hours.

Causes / Contributing factors

- PRCV is respiratory spread.
- Believed to be windborne long distances.

Diagnosis

PRCV does however cross react with the serological test for TGE and it therefore can confuse the diagnosis. A differential test is available but recently this has failed suggesting a new or different virus has appeared. In such infected herds respiratory disease is becoming evident particularly in the presence of PRRS virus.

Treatment

- There is no specific treatment.
- Use broad spectrum antibiotics in feed, water or by injection. Including tetracyclines and trimethoprim/sulpha.

Porcine Stress Syndrome (PSS)

(Chapter 9 pp326)

This term covers several conditions associated with an autosomal recessive gene. It includes acute stress and sudden death (malignant hyperthermia), pale soft exudative muscle (PSE), dark firm dry meat, and back muscle necrosis. Heavy muscled pigs are more likely to carry the gene.

The pig is either homozygous (susceptible), heterozygous or free of the gene (both non susceptible). The gene can be identified by the pigs response to the anaesthetic gas halothane but recent developments have produced gene probes using blood or hair, that identify both the homozygous and heterozygous carriers.

When the homozygous state is present and following a period of muscle activity, there is a change in muscle metabolism from aerobic to anaerobic and biochemical abnormalities develop. The body tissues become acid with a marked rise in temperature 42ºC (107ºF).

Symptoms

- ☞ The onset is sudden with muscle tremors.
- ☞ Twitching of the face
- ☞ Rapid respiration.
- ☞ The skin becomes red and blotched.
- ☞ Death usually occurs within 15-20 minutes.
- ☞ Back muscle necrosis is a more localised form of PSS.
- ☞ Whilst the gene produces a leaner carcass, growth rates are slower and the levels of sudden death increase.

Causes / Contributing factors

- ◆ Disease is precipitated by sudden muscle activity.
- ◆ The carrier pig is genetically susceptible.

Diagnosis

This is based on the sudden onset, symptoms, breed, susceptibility and the known presence or absence of the gene in the pig. In many cases the pig is just found dead and a post-mortem examination is necessary to eliminate other disease. Rigor mortis (stiffening of the muscles after death) within 5 minutes is a striking feature.

This condition has to be differentiated from other causes of sudden death, twisted bowel, internal haemorrhage, mulberry heart disease and pyelonephritis.

Treatment

Treatment is usually ineffective but the following are worth trying:

- ❒ Spray the pig with cold water to control the temperature rises.
- ❒ Inject 50-100ml of calcium gluconate (used in cows for milk fever) by intramuscular injections at two separate sites. Seek veterinary advice.
- ❒ Sedate the pig with stresnil.
- ❒ Do not move or cause undue muscle activity.
- ❒ Give an injection of vitamin E, 2iu/kg.

Prolapse of the Rectum

(Chapter 9 pp327)

This is a widespread condition occurring in growing pigs from 8 to 20 weeks of age. The onset is sudden.

Symptoms

- ☞ The size of the prolapse varies from 10 to 80mm and if small it will often revert into the rectum spontaneously.
- ☞ In most cases however the prolapse remains out becomes swollen and filled with fluid.
- ☞ It is also prone to damage with haemorrhage.
- ☞ Cannibalism often results by other pigs in the pen as shown by blood on the noses of the offending pigs and on the flanks of others.
- ☞ Blown up abdomen seen in pigs 2 - 4 weeks after prolapse (rectal stricture).
- ☞ Pale pigs due to haemorrhage.
- ☞ Sometimes death.

Causes / Contributing factors

- The fundamental cause is an increase in abdominal pressure which forces the rectum to the exterior and a swelling of the mucous lining and then straining.

The following may be considered as causal or contributory.

- Diarrhoea - excessive straining.
- Respiratory disease - excessive coughing increasing abdominal pressure.
- Colitis - abnormal fermentation occurs in the large bowel with

the production of excessive gas increasing abdominal pressure.

- In cold weather the incidence of rectal prolapses increases. This is associated with low house temperatures and the tendency of pigs to huddle together, thus increasing abdominal pressure.
- Wet conditions and slippery floors, particularly those with no bedding, increase abdominal pressure.
- If stocking densities reach the level whereby pigs cannot lay out on their sides across the pen the incidence may increase. It is often related to specific houses on the farm.
- Nutrition
    - Ad lib feeding - Feeding pigs to appetite results in continual heavy gut fill and indigestion. There is then a tendency for abnormal fermentation in the large bowel because undigest ed components of the feed arrive in greater amounts.
    - High density diets and in particular lysine levels increase growth rates and outbreaks may often subside either by a change to restricted feeding or using a lower energy / lysine diet.
    - Water shortage - This can lead to constipation.
    - Diets high in starch may predispose to prolapse - Try adding 2-4% grass meal to the diet.
    - The presence of mycotoxins in feed - If there is a problem make sure that the bins have been well cleaned out. Examine the cereal sources.
    - Change of diet - By studying the timing of the problem it is sometimes possible to identify rectal prolapses not only with a change of diet but also a change of housing.
    - Trauma
    - Tail docking - docking tails too short can damage the nerve supply to the anal ring leading to a relaxation of the anal sphincter.

Diagnosis

This is based on the clinical picture.

Treatment

❒ Rectal prolapses must be recognised early and the pig removed from the pen.

- Replace the prolapse and retain it by a purse string or mattress suture. Return the pig to the pen. The technique for carrying this out is described in *Chapter 15 pp 501*.
- In some cases the prolapse will be completely bitten off by other pigs. Here the pig should be left in the pen as most cases will progress to slaughter although a few will develop rectal strictures. Here the rectum closes up the pigs cannot pass faeces and the abdomen swells up. Destroy such pigs.

Collect the following information about each prolapse to see if common factors emerge:

Age of pig.
Comments observations.
Days in the house.
Diet fed.
House type and pen.
Number of pigs per pen
Number of rectal strictures.
Number of prolapses sutured.
Outcome.
State of prolapse.
Tail biting.
Weight of the pig.

Rabies

This is similar in all pigs see Section 2.

Rectal Stricture

(Chapter 9 pp328)

This is a condition often considered a sequel to rectal prolapse. Approximately a fingers length inside the rectum the tissues gradually shrink, scar tissue develops and eventually the tube completely closes. The area where the stricture occurs is supplied by two tiny arteries that originate from the aorta. Some studies suggest that if these arteries are blocked or thrombosed by bacteria a rectal stricture will result. Erysipelas, *Haemophilus parasuis*, streptococci and salmonella have been implicated.

Symptoms

Affected pigs in the early stage of the disease often show:

- ☞ A very loose diarrhoea that becomes projectile.
- ☞ A gradual increase in the size of the abdomen.
- ☞ Loss of condition.

Causes / Contributing factors

- ◆ Infection and thrombosis of blood vessels.
- ◆ Sequel to rectal prolapse.

Diagnosis

Based on clinical signs.

Treatment

- ❐ There is no treatment for this condition and as soon as pigs are recognised they should be destroyed on welfare grounds. Attempting to open up the stricture by palpation has in the author's experience been a total failure.
- ❐ If rectal strictures occur in large numbers at predictable times consider infection as a cause and assess the effects of strategic medication by injection, water or in-feed.

Rotavirus Infection

(Chapter 9 pp333)

These viruses are widespread in mammals. They are present in most pig herds with 100% sero-conversion in adult stock. They persist outside the pig, where they are resistant to environmental changes and many disinfectants. Maternal antibodies last for 3-6 weeks after which pigs become susceptible to infection but exposure does not necessarily result in disease. It is estimated that only 10-15% of diarrhoea in pigs is initiated by a primary rotavirus infection.

Symptoms

In a mature herd:

- ☞ A watery profuse diarrhoea appears after piglets are 7 to 10 days of age. It becomes progressively less important with age.

- ☞ However if pathogenic strains of *E. coli* are present severe disease can occur with heavy mortality.
- ☞ Villus atrophy is a consistent feature which results in malabsorption.
- ☞ Dehydration.
- ☞ Diarrhoea usually lasts 3-4 days.
- ☞ Pigs look hollow.
- ☞ Eyes are sunken.
- ☞ Skin around the rectum is wet.

The role of rotaviruses in the post-weaned pig is probably less important although they are often identified when acute *E. coli* diarrhoea occurs in the first 7-10 days after weaning.

Causes / Contributing factors

- Poor house hygiene.
- Permanently populated houses.
- Movement of pigs.
- Temperature fluctuations.
- Contaminated boots and clothing.

Diagnosis

Whenever there is a diarrhoea problem in pigs between 10 and 40 days of age rotavirus infection either as primary agents or secondary must be considered. Electron microscopy and ELISA tests in the laboratory are required for confirmation. Try the litmus test by soaking scour in litmus paper, *E. coli* infections turn blue, virus infections red.

Treatment

- ❒ There are no specific treatments for rotavirus infections.
- ❒ Provide antibiotic therapy either by injection, by mouth or in the drinking water, to control secondary infections such as *E. coli.*
- ❒ Apralan, amoxycillin, neomycin, framycetin and enrofloxacin could be used.
- ❒ Provide dextrose/glycine electrolytes to counteract dehydration. *(Chapter 14 pp 127)*
- ❒ Provide dry warm and comfortable lying areas.

Ruptures or Hernias

(Chapter 9 pp334)

Of many congenital abnormalities, umbilical or inguinal ruptures are most common. They are considered to be developmental defects and have a very low heritability. Umbilical hernias can sometimes be traced back to a particular boar in which case he should be culled.

Symptoms

- ☞ Swellings 30 - 200mm in diameter protruding from the umbilicus and abdomen, or below and in front of the testicles or in the groin (inguinal rupture).
- ☞ If the swellings are large trauma to the skin may cause ulcerations particularly umbilical ruptures.

Causes / Contributing factors

Environmental factors can increase the incidence of umbilical hernias so if there is a problem (more than 2% of pigs) consider the following:

- Are prostaglandins used to synchronise farrowings. If so check that piglets are not being pulled away from the sow at farrowing and the cord stretched excessively.
- Is navel bleeding occurring on the farm? Are naval clips being used to prevent bleeding? If so make sure they are not placed close up to the skin otherwise the tissues will be damaged and weakened.
- Identify the precise time when the ruptures appear. Do these coincide with a change of housing?
- In housing where the pigs pass through a small hole to the dunging area sudden severe abdominal pressure may cause ruptures.
- Are stocking densities high and causing increased abdominal pressure?
- In cold weather do the pigs huddle thereby increasing abdominal pressure?
- Check records to see if any particular boar is implicated.
- If the rupture is large and the pig is on a concrete floor or slats it should be moved to a soft bedded area so that the overlying

skin does not become sore and ulcerated.

- Examine navels at births and two days later to see if there are any abnormalities.

Diagnosis

Visual evidence. Reduction of the bowel contents in the rupture when squeezed back into the abdomen.

Treatment

- Inguinal ruptures are not as important a problem unless they become very large. Where castration is the farm policy a minor surgical operation needs to be performed. This is described in *chapter 15* of the main manual.
- Sometimes peritonitis results. Destruction may be necessary.

SALMONELLOSIS

(Chapter 9 pp334)

Of the many serotypes of salmonella that exist, the ones that are most likely to cause clinical disease in pigs are *Salmonella choleraesuis*, and *Salmonella typhimurium* and to a lesser extent *Salmonella derby*. Other "exotic" salmonella serotypes may infect pigs and be shed in the faeces for limited periods but they usually remain sub-clinical. *S. choleraesuis* and *S. derby* are the specific host-adapted pig serovars. *S. choleraesuis* can cause major generalised disease. *S. typhimurium* and *S. derby* are more likely to cause milder disease the main sign of which is usually diarrhoea. Pigs may become long-term sub-clinical carriers of *S. choleraesuis* and *S. derby,* the organisms surviving in the mesenteric lymph nodes draining the intestine. Many such carriers do not shed the bacteria in faeces unless they are stressed. Pigs may be intermittent or continuous faecal shedders of other serotypes but the carrier state is usually short, weeks or a few months and is self limiting. Remember that *S. typhimurium,* which occasionally can be isolated from pigs, are common causes of food poisoning in people.

Salmonellosis can occur at any age but is most common in growing pigs over eight weeks of age. Severe *S. choleraesuis* infection occurs typically at around 12 to 14 weeks.

Symptoms

- ☞ The acute septicaemia and pneumonia which may occur with *S. choleraesuis* may result in fever, inappetence, respiratory distress, depression, coughing and poor doing pigs.
- ☞ The skin of the extremities (i.e. tail, ears, nose and feet) become blue.
- ☞ Foul-smelling diarrhoea which may be blood stained, is a common feature.
- ☞ Yellow jaundice may result from liver damage and lameness from arthritis.
- ☞ Nervous signs resulting from meningitis.
- ☞ If untreated, mortality may be high.
- ☞ Infections with *S. typhimurium* usually are manifest by diarrhoea.

Causes / Contributing factors

- Poor hygiene.
- Overcrowding.
- Stress by moving and mixing.
- Permanently populated houses.
- Contaminated boots and clothing.
- Mechanical means via faeces and the movement of contaminated equipment.
- Vermin and flies.
- Contamination of feed by birds, rats and mice
- Contamination of raw feed ingredients and thus the final product.

Diagnosis

The post-mortem lesions are strongly suggestive of *S. choleraesuis*, particularly the generalised pneumonia, the appearance of the lining of the small and large intestine, the congested spleen and multiple small haemorrhages. However, to make a specific diagnosis it is necessary to submit to the laboratory either fresh faecal samples from untreated pigs or where available a dead or live untreated pig.

Severe salmonellosis caused by *S. choleraesuis* can occur alone but it also commonly occurs with classical swine fever (hog cholera) in those countries in which this disease still occurs. In such countries it is important to ensure by serology and laboratory tests that swine fever is not the primary cause (NB. swine fever usually also affects sows and sucking piglets and also causes mummified litters and abortions).

Severe PRRS in herds with endemic EP may give the appearance of salmonellosis, however PRRS also causes abortions, stillbirths and precipitates scouring in piglets.

Treatment

- ❐ The response to treatment is often poor. It is helpful to determine the antibiotic sensitivity and treat individual pigs at a very early stage.
- ❐ Note that some veterinarians disagree with the treating of salmonellosis and advocate only improved hygiene and lowered stocking densities.
- ❐ Strategic medication in-feed or in the water can be effective. The drugs used are based on the bacterial sensitivity.

The severity of clinical salmonellosis is dose dependant. The overall aim, therefore, is to get the levels in the environment down to below the disease-producing threshold. The second aim is to reduce the spread of infection.

Remember that salmonella can cause disease in people and is one of the commonest causes of food poisoning. This has two implications for you as a pig farmer. First, you should ensure that everybody working with the pigs adopts a high standard of personal hygiene so that they do not become infected. Second, it is important that pig farmers and pig meat products have a high public image for safety and do not get linked with outbreaks of human disease. It is therefore imperative that you get salmonella under strict control.

Salt Poisoning - Water Deprivation

(Chapter 9 pp336)

Salt poisoning is common in all ages of pigs and is related to water shortage either caused by inadequate supplies or complete loss of supply. It should be a daily routine to check that all sources of water are adequate, free flowing and available. The normal levels of salt in the diet (0.4-0.5%) become toxic in the absence of water.

Symptoms

- ☞ The very early stages of disease are preceded by inappetence. Whenever a sow or group of pigs are not eating always check the water supply first. Signs develop within 24 to 48 hours.
- ☞ The first signs are often pigs trying to drink from nipple drinkers unsuccessfully.
- ☞ Nervous signs then develop with fits and animals wandering around apparently blind, trembling and incoordinated.
- ☞ Often the pig walks up to a wall, stands and presses its head against it.
- ☞ One sign strongly suggestive of salt poisoning is dog sitting and nose twitching just before a convulsion starts and jerky eye movements.

Causes / Contributing factors

- Water shortage/deprivation.
- Excess salt in the diet.

Diagnosis

This is based upon the clinical signs and lack of water. Examination of the brain histologically at post-mortem confirms the disease.

Salt poisoning must be distinguished from Aujeszky's disease (pseudorabies), swine fever, streptococcal meningitis and glässers disease which all produce nervous signs. It might also be confused with middle ear infection but this only affects one individual rather than a group of pigs.

Treatment

- ❐ The response to treatment is poor and involves rehydrating the animal. At a practical level this can be achieved by dripping water into the mouth of the pig through a hose pipe or alternatively via a flutter valve into the rectum where it is absorbed. (See *Chapter 15 pp 486* "Flutter valve").
- ❐ Discuss the possibility of administering sterile water into the abdomen with your veterinarian.
- ❐ Corticosteroids may also help.

Spirochaetal Diarrhoea

(Chapter 9 pp336)

This is a disease associated with spirochetes distinct from the one that cause swine dysentery. It occurs mainly in growing pigs appearing very similar to non-specific colitis and PIA caused by *Lawsonia intracellularis*. Spirochetes are common inhabitants of the large intestine and caecum.

Symptoms

☞ A mild to moderate diarrhoea develops two to six weeks post-weaning that persists for a few days.

☞ Dehydration.

☞ Loss in growth.

☞ Most cases resolve in 7 to 10 days but in some pigs it becomes chronic.

☞ The disease can be difficult to differentiate from other bacterial infections, particularly non-specific colitis.

Causes / Contributing factors

- A sudden change in diet.
- Removal of copper from the diet.
- Withdrawal of growth promoters.
- Poor hygiene i.e. dirty floor surfaces, water contamination.

Diagnosis

This is difficult because specific organisms cannot usually be identified. If there is an on-going problem on the farm, live diseased pigs showing typical signs, should be submitted for post-mortem and bacteriological examinations to eliminate swine dysentery.

Treatment

❐ In-feed medication with lincomycin, tiamulin (monensin, dimetridazole if available) or tylosin can be used effectively for both prevention and treatment.

❐ In acute outbreaks lincomycin, tiamulin or tylosin could be given in the water.

❐ Inject individual pigs with either lincomycin, tiamulin or tylosin and assess the response.

Streptococcal Infections

(Chapter 9 pp336)

Streptococci are common organisms in all animals. They are broadly but not entirely species specific. The main species in pigs is *Streptococcus suis* which is widespread in pig populations and probably occurs wherever pig farming is carried out. It is associated with a variety of conditions including meningitis, septicaemia, polyserisitis, arthritis, endocarditis and pneumonia. It has also been isolated from cases of rhinitis and abortion. The pattern and relative importance of the different syndromes vary in different countries.

S. suis is sub-divided into at least thirty-four serotypes. They vary in their pathogenicity and the clinical signs they cause, both between and within types. Some types appear to be non-pathogenic and have been isolated mainly from healthy pigs, some are mainly associated with lung lesions, and some have been isolated from other animal species as well as pigs. Some types, mainly 2, can occasionally cause meningitis in people as well as pigs. Fortunately human cases are rare.

The syndrome that is important and worrying to the pig farmer is persistent endemic meningitis caused by type 2.

Clinically healthy pigs can carry the organism in their tonsils for many months and a carrier state exists in some sows. Once a serotype has entered a herd no techniques are yet available to remove it and it becomes established as part of the normal flora. *S. suis* is quickly killed by disinfectants in common use on farms, including phenolic disinfectants and chlorine and iodine based ones. Detergents will also kill the organism in thirty minutes. 'Savlon ' is particularly effective. Outside the pig, in very cold and freezing conditions, it may survive for 15 weeks or more but at normal room temperatures it dies within one to two weeks. It survives long periods in rotting carcasses.

The sow passes on antibody through colostrum to the sucking pig and the disease is therefore uncommon in this group of animals unless it is introduced into the herd for the first time. It is much more common in the immediate post-weaning period often starting

2 to 3 weeks after weaning and continuing through to approximately 16 weeks of age. In flat decks or nurseries almost 100% of pigs become carriers within three weeks.

There are also strains of low pathogenicity which may be activated by PRRS virus infection. PRRS may also raise the incidence of meningitis caused by pathogenic strains when it first enters a herd. Although PRRS alone does not affect the brain, it has been shown experimentally that many more pigs are affected with meningitis when they are infected with both *S. suis* type 2 and PRRS viruses than when they are infected with *S. suis* alone. *S. suis* type 14 which was first isolated from a case of human meningitis is emerging as a new disease in the UK with the appearance of acute severe outbreaks of arthritis in both sucking and weaned pigs.

Species of streptococci other than *S. suis* may sometimes cause disease in pigs. For example, *Streptococcus equisimilis* causes sporadic cases of septicaemia and arthritis in sucking pigs, infection of the heart valves in growing pigs and ascending infection of the womb in sows. In the USA *Streptococcus porcinus* causes throat abscesses and septicaemia and is sometimes isolated from pneumonia. However, cases of streptococcal throat abscesses have become rare in modern systems of pig housing.

Symptoms

Cases of acute type 2 meningitis:

- The pig may just be found dead.
- In very early stages of meningitis the pig is laid on its belly, hair standing on end and shivering.
- Within two to three hours there are lateral jerky movements of the eye (nystagmus).
- The animal then lies on its side paddling and frothing at the mouth.
- The organism invades the blood stream and is carried around the body where it may cause arthritis and pneumonia.
- Severe arthritis, pigs squeal with pain and refuse to stand.

Type 1 occurs fairly commonly in most countries and causes:

- Sporadic arthritis.

Occasionally meningitis is seen in sucking piglets usually around one to two weeks of age but sometimes up to six weeks. It is a relatively unimportant condition.

Causes / Contributing factors

- *S. suis* is spread from one pig to another by direct nose to nose contact.
- Carrier boars or gilts.
- It can also spread within a herd by indirect contact.
- In confined space by aerosol infection.

If you have the disease endemic in your herd the incidence increases with :-

- High stocking density in flat decks.
- Continuous production systems which perpetuate infection.
- Concurrent PRRS infections.
- Mixing of pigs post-weaning.
- Too small cubic capacity air space per pig. Provide at least $0.8m^3$ per pig at weaning.
- Poor ventilation and high humidity.
- High dust levels.
- Stress.
- Damp pens.
- High slurry levels under perforated metal floors.
- Weighing pigs and associated stress.
- Tattooing, ear notching and extra stress at weaning.
- Changes in nutritional status at critical times.
- Low vitamin E in the diet. Assess the response to adding 50-100iu/kg.

Diagnosis

A history of the presence of recurring meningitis in weaned pigs is highly suggestive and is confirmed by the isolation of the organism from the brain and its specific identification, which not all diagnostic laboratories are capable of.

Because of the existence of strains that are non-pathogenic or only mildly pathogenic, the isolation of *S. suis* type 2 from the tonsils of a pig is difficult to interpret. Isolation from the brain of a pig showing signs of meningitis is more conclusive.

The disease must be differentiated from aujeszky's disease, glässers disease or salt poisoning (water deprivation) which all produce nervous signs.

Treatment

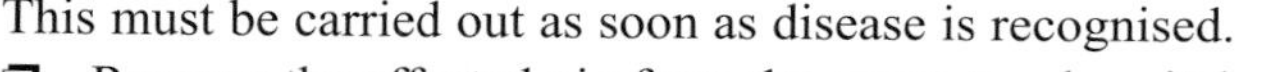

This must be carried out as soon as disease is recognised.

- ❒ Remove the affected pig from the group to a hospital pen.
- ❒ The recovery rate is increased substantially through good nursing. Provide warmth and bedding and trickle water into the pigs mouth from a hosepipe every 4 to 6 hours. Alternatively, water can be given by inserting a narrow hosepipe gently into the pigs rectum or using a flutter valve. *(See Chapter 15).*
- ❒ Give intra-muscular injections of penicillin 2 to 3 times daily for the first 24 hours.
- ❒ Use a quick acting penicillin for the first 24 hours followed by long-acting penicillin. Time is of the essence with this disease.

Strategic medication is a method to adopt on farms where disease levels remain high. The following options are available:

- ❒ Identify the onset of disease and apply strategic medication 2 to 3 days before that time.
- ❒ Strategic medication can be applied in the drinking water using phenoxymethyl penicillin, tetracyclines, synthetic penicillin particularly amoxycillin, or trimethoprim/sulpha.
- ❒ In-feed medicate continuously from day of weaning through to six weeks post-weaning. Phenoxymethyl penicillin at a level of 300g/tonne is the drug of choice. TMS could also be used.
- ❒ Inject all pigs with long-acting penicillin at weaning time.

Sunburn

This is similar in all pigs see Section 2.

Swine Dysentery (SD)

(Chapter 9 pp338)

Swine dysentery (SD), is caused by a spirochaetal bacterium called *Serpulina hyodysenteriae*. Disease is common in pigs from

12 to 75kg but severe cases occur occasionally in sows and their sucking piglets.

SD will survive outside the pig for up to seven weeks in cold moist conditions but it dies out in two days in dry warm environments.

Spread through the herd is slow, building up in numbers as the dose rate of the causal agent builds up in the environment. Pigs that recover develop a low immunity and rarely suffer from the disease again.

The high cost of disease is associated with mortality (low), morbidity (high), depression of growth and feed conversion efficiency, and costs of continual in-feed medication.

The incubation period in field cases is normally 7 to 14 days but can be as long as 60 days. Pigs may develop a sub-clinical carrier state initially and then break down with clinical disease when put under stress or when there is a change of feed.

Symptoms

The first signs are:

- ☞ Sloppy diarrhoea, which stains the skin under the anus.
- ☞ Initially the diarrhoea is light brown and contains jelly-like mucus.
- ☞ Twitching of the tail.
- ☞ Hollowing of the flanks.
- ☞ Partial loss of appetite.
- ☞ Slight reddening of the skin.

As the disease progresses:

- ☞ Blood may appear in increasing amounts turning the faeces dark and tarry.
- ☞ The pig rapidly loses condition.
- ☞ Becomes dehydrated.
- ☞ A gaunt appearance with sunken eyes.
- ☞ Sudden death sometimes occurs mainly in heavy finishers.

Causes / Contributing factors

- Pigs become infected through the ingestion of infected faeces.
- Spread is by carrier pigs that shed the organism in faeces for long periods.

- It may enter the farm through the introduction of carrier pigs.
- Mechanically in infected faeces via equipment, contaminated delivery pipe of feed vehicles, boots or birds.
- It can be spread by flies, mice, birds and dogs.
- Stress resulting from change of feed may precipitate.
- Poor sanitation and wet pens enhance the disease.
- Overcrowding.

Diagnosis

This is based on the history, the clinical picture, post-mortem examinations, laboratory tests on faecal smears and the isolation and identification of *S. hyodysenteriae* by serological and biochemical tests and DNA analysis. Identification requires specialised procedures which are not available in every laboratory.

Post-mortem examinations show that the lesions are confined to the large bowel and sometimes the greater curvature of the stomach.

The disease has to be distinguished from colitis caused by other spirochetes, non-specific colitis, PIA and bloody gut (PHE), acute salmonella infections and heavy infections of the whip worm, trichuris.

Treatment

- ❒ The following drugs can be used in treatment:

Carbadox. *	Ronidazol.e *
Dimetridazole. *	Salinomycin.
Tiamulin.	Lincomycin.
Tylosin.	Monensin. *

  (* may not be available)

  Some strains of *S. hyodysenteriae* have become resistant to some of these drugs.
- ❒ With the first signs of disease medicate the drinking water with either lincomycin, tiamulin or tylosin for at least 7 days.
- ❒ Inject badly affected individual pigs daily for 4 days with lincomycin, tiamulin or tylosin.
- ❒ In-feed medication is only of value in preventing clinical disease developing.

Eradication

There are two broad options which should be discussed with your veterinarian, either depopulate and repopulate with clean pigs or attempt to eradicate the disease without depopulation. Be aware that they are both expensive and the success rate is not 100% particularly with the second option.

In the farrow to finish herd, eradication without depopulation starts with the treatment of the sows and sucking piglets to provide *S. hyodysenteriae* free weaners. Such pigs must not be allowed to come into contact with any other infected pigs or their faeces. There are a number of programmes that can be adopted .
The following drugs and regimes have been used successfully for the eradication of swine dysentery.

<u>Sows:</u>
Period of medication up to 8 weeks.
Dimetridazole 500 to 800g/tonne feed.
Tiamulin 100g/tonne feed.
Lincomycin 110g/tonne feed.
Monensin 100g/tonne feed.

<u>Weaners:</u>
Period of in-feed medication three weeks.
Lincomycin 110-220g/tonne of creep feed.
Tiamulin 100g/tonne of creep feed.

<u>Growers:</u>
Lincomycin 55 to 110 g/tonne.
Tiamulin 60 to 100 g/tonne.
Monensin 100 g/tonne.

If you are successful in eradicating swine dysentery take strict precautions not to let it re-enter your herd. Transmission usually requires a largish dose of infected faeces so the disease can be kept out even in pig dense areas.

Swine Fevers
African Swine Fever(ASF)
Classical Swine Fever(CSF) also known as Hog Cholera (HC)

(Chapter 12 pp403)

Swine fever is one of the most important virus diseases of pigs. It is notifiable in most countries of the world. Control is by slaughter or as a last resort by vaccination. African swine fever (ASF) and Classical Swine fever are caused by very similar viruses which are only distinguishable by laboratory testing. Both are dealt with in *Chapter 12.*

Symptoms

☞ Pigs dejected - hang their heads.
☞ Not eating.
☞ Pigs chilled - huddled together.
☞ Diarrhoea.
☞ Eye discharge - heavy.
☞ High persistent fever.
☞ Nervous signs - Incoordination, swaying on the legs.
☞ Blue discoloration of the skin.
☞ High mortality.

Causes / Contributing factors

◆ Transmitted via infected frozen or uncooked pork.

Diagnosis

This is based on the symptoms, rapid spread and very ill pigs. Laboratory tests are used to confirm disease.

Treatment

❐ None.

Swine Influenza Virus (SI)

(Chapter 9 pp341)

In the pig there are at least four different serotypes of the virus each stimulating immunity to itself but not to the other serotypes. It is thus possible for the pigs to be infected by each one sequentially or at the same time. Clinical outbreaks usually occur in the winter although the virus may remain circulating sub-clinically or with sporadic minor episodes in the herd throughout the rest of the year. The incubation period is short, less than 48 hours and the onset is usually rapid and dramatic. It is virtually impossible to maintain a population of pigs that is influenza virus free.

Symptoms

Acute disease:

- ☞ Classically the pigs suddenly become prostrate.
- ☞ Breathing heavily.
- ☞ Severe coughing.
- ☞ Most of them look as if they are going to die but most of them survive without treatment unless the herd already has a respiratory disease problem.
- ☞ SI causes severe pneumonia on its own but when it is combined with other infections such as App, EP and PRRS an intractable chronic respiratory disease syndrome can develop. Severely affected individuals or groups of pigs are therefore best given antibiotic cover to prevent secondary pneumonias developing.

Endemic disease:

- ☞ Here the virus remains in the herd, affecting small groups of pigs often weaners. It may be responsible for continuing respiratory diseases with symptoms as in acute disease but less dramatic.

Causes / Contributing factors

- The virus can be transmitted between people, pigs and birds, particularly water fowl, by direct contact or aerosol.
- Poor environment, poor ventilation increase the severity of disease.

Diagnosis

Diagnosis of classical acute disease is based on the rapidity of development and spread, together with typical clinical signs. No other disease affects so many pigs so quickly. In the chronic respiratory disease syndrome it is necessary to carry out serological tests and/or virus isolation to determine the presence and type of virus.

Treatment

- ❒ Control secondary bacterial pneumonias with antibiotics.
- ❒ Treat severely affected pigs by injection.
- ❒ Medicate the water for 3 - 5 days.
- ❒ Use OTC, CTC, tiamulin, lincomycin or trimethoprim/sulpha.

Swine Pox

(Chapter 10 pp363)

This is a disease caused by the swine pox virus which can survive outside the pig for long periods of time and is resistant to environmental changes. It is a vesicular disease.

Symptoms

- ☞ Small circular red areas 10-20mm in diameter that commence with a vesicle containing straw-coloured fluid in the centre.
- ☞ After two to three days the vesicle ruptures and a scab is formed which gradually turns black.
- ☞ The lesions may be seen on any part of the body but are common along the flanks, abdomens and occasionally the ears.

Causes / Contributing factors

- ◆ It can be spread by lice or mange mites.
- ◆ Skin abrasions.
- ◆ Fighting and mixing of pigs.

Diagnosis

It can be confused with localised greasy pig disease, pustular dermatitis and the allergic form of mange. Close examination shows swine pox lesions.

Treatment

- ❒ There is no treatment and the condition usually resolves itself spontaneously over a three week period.

Swine Vesicular Disease (SVD)

(See Chapter 12 pp411)

Although the virus that causes swine vesicular disease (SVD) is different from that causing foot and mouth disease (FMD) it produces a disease in pigs that is clinically indistinguishable from FMD.

This disease should always be considered if sudden widespread lameness appears with vesicles or blisters on the snout, tongue and tops of the claws. In most countries it is notifiable and if suspected must be reported to the authorities immediately.

TETANUS

This is similar in all pigs see Section 2.

TORSION OF THE STOMACH AND INTESTINES

(Chapter 9 pp341)

This is a common cause of sudden death in the growing pig and often affects one of the best pigs in the group. It also occurs in sows and occasionally piglets.

Symptoms

☞ Usually none but sudden death.
☞ Grossly distended abdomen.
☞ The carcass is fresh but the pig is very pale.

Causes / Contributing factors

- Deaths are usually sporadic although they can be of significance where, for example, whey is being fed and bloat occurs.
- Over-feeding and abnormal fermentation of the contents of both the small and large intestine result in gas formation, increased pressure and torsion.
- Prolonged over excitement at feeding may predispose.

Diagnosis

Post-mortem examination shows the small and large intestines heavily congested and full of blood. The intestinal tract in the pig is suspended from a common point and this makes it liable to rotate and twist.

Treatment

❒ Mortality in weaned and growing pigs should normally be less than 3% but up to a third of this may be caused by torsion. If it reaches 1% or more the dietary components should be examined closely to see if there are starch based ingredients that might cause excessive fermentation. In such cases increasing the level of the growth promoter (if allowed) or by adding 100g/tonne of penicillin, OTC or tylosin should reduce the bacterial multiplication.

If torsion is a consistent cause of death collect information about each case including weight, age, sex, house, stocking density, environmental temperatures and feed changes. A study of this may give guidance as to contributing causes.

Transmissible Gastro-Enteritis (TGE)

(See Section 2 and *Chapter 9 pp 342)*

This is a highly infectious disease which in the weaning and the growing pig is clinically indistinguishable from porcine epidemic diarrhoea. In small grower-finisher units the virus is likely to disappear from the population. In large finishing units in which susceptible pigs are being brought in frequently, the virus is maintained indefinitely in the population by repeated infection of the newcomers.

Symptoms

- ☞ When the virus is introduced into a finishing herd for the first time there is rapidly spreading, vomiting and a watery diarrhoea, eventually affecting almost all the animals.
- ☞ Disease disappears spontaneously over a 3 to 5 week period.
- ☞ Mortality is usually low.
- ☞ The main effect on the individual growing pig is dehydration which is resolved in about a week.
- ☞ Nevertheless the disease may increase the slaughter age by 5-10 days.

Causes / Contributing factors

- Continual use of buildings without all-in, all-out may perpetuate disease.
- Continual purchase of naive weaners.

Diagnosis

This is based on the clinical symptoms and high mortality with acute, severe diarrhoea in sucking pigs (if present).

Treatment

- ❒ There is no treatment.

- ❐ Provide electrolytes and easy access to water to prevent dehydration.
- ❐ Maintain warm dry environments during acute disease.

The virus is sensitive to ultra violet radiation and in warm temperatures will only survive outside the pig for a few days. If an endemic situation therefore develops on a farrow-to-finish farm make a minimum break of 3 weeks in summer time by segregated disease control of the nurseries, together with clean up and disinfection, to break the cycle of infection. Alternatively if pigs are being brought into a finishing unit frequently, make a break of 3 or 4 weeks.

TUBERCULOSIS

(Chapter 9 pp342)

Tuberculosis affects mammals, including people, and birds. The causal organism, *Mycobacterium tuberculosis*, is sub-classified into types, human, bovine and avian. The avian type is referred to as *M. avium* or more often the *avian/intracellulare* complex because it is not a uniform species. *M. avium* itself infects mainly birds but is also found in the environment along with *M. intracellulare* which is predominantly saprophytic or free living. Pigs are rarely infected by the human or bovine types but are commonly infected by the avian/intracellulare complex.

The *avian/intracellulare* complex also causes sub-clinical non-progressive infection in healthy people. The main concern is that it could cause more serious disease in immuno-suppressed people and people with AIDS.

In most countries if lesions are found in the neck at slaughter the whole head is condemned and if they are found in the mesenteric lymph nodes which drain the intestines the offals are condemned. If they are more widespread in the body, which is rare, the whole carcass may be condemned or cooked. If small lesions are missed by the meat inspector normal kitchen cooking destroys the organism.

Symptoms

- ☞ It causes small nodules in the lymph nodes of the neck and those that drain the small intestine.

☞ In the great majority of cases the lesions are non-progressive, they do not spread through the body, do not make the pig ill and are not excreted.

☞ There are no clinical symptoms and there is no difference in performance between infected and non-infected pigs.

Causes / Contributing factors

- The disease does not spread between pigs and should be regarded as an environmental infection. It is rarely diagnosed in living pigs.
- Paddocks that have been treated with poultry manure up to one year previously, (or, in the case of bovine TB, which have been grazed by infected cattle or badgers).
- Avian TB as the name implies is found in wild birds. The organism is shed in large numbers via droppings and therefore food, grain or bedding contaminated by birds becomes a potent source.
- Peat often contains *M. intracellulare*. Peat is used both for bedding and gut stimulation in the young piglets. It should only be used if it as been pasteurised.
- Water contaminated by *M. avium/intracellulare* is often a source.

Diagnosis

In living pigs diagnosis is by the skin tuberculin test but usually it is brought to the farmer's attention by high condemnation rates at slaughter.

Treatment

❐ There is no treatment.

Vice - Abnormal Behaviour

(Chapter 9 pp343)

Vice can be a major problem with considerable economic loss. Why do pigs mutilate each other? Poor environmental conditions and poor stockmanship cause aggravation and aggression. Stand for a few minutes and observe pigs that are either tail biting or ear chewing and you will see that there is one overriding feature, the pigs give the impression of being very unhappy. If you notice that only one pig appears to be the aggressor, remove it from the pen.

Types of Vice

The weaned pig	Growers
Penis / navel sucking.	Tail biting.
Prepuce sucking.	Ear necrosis.
Ear sucking.	Chewing feet.
Tail biting.	Flank biting.

Symptoms

- Evident by trauma and infection of the skin.
- Lameness.
- Mortality.

Causes / Contributing factors

- Management factors
  - A change in the diet.
  - Long tails.
  - Draughts.
  - Fluctuating temperatures.
  - High air speed .
  - High stocking densities.
  - Shortage of trough space.
  - Ammonia levels > 20ppm.
  - A very humid environment.
  - Aggressive breeds.
  - No bedding.
  - Trauma.
  - Uncomfortable conditions.
  - Unhappy pigs.
  - Water shortage.
  - Wet pens.
  - Automatic feeding and little human/pig empathy.
  - High hydrogen sulphide levels > 10ppm.
  - Pigs too small for the environment.
  - Bad pen designs - badly sited feeders.
  - High carbon dioxide levels > 3000ppm.
- Nutritional factors
  - Low salt in the diet.
  - Diet changes.
  - Feeding pellets.
  - Inadequate nutrition.
  - Poor feed availability.
  - Rations with small particle sizes.
- Disease factors
  - Wet eczema.
  - PRRS skin lesions.
  - Swine pox.
  - Pneumonia.
  - Greasy pig disease.
  - New concrete and skin trauma.
  - Colitis.
  - Skin trauma.
  - Parasites.

Diagnosis

Based on observations and skin lesions.

Treatment

- ❒ If *Staphylococcus hyicus* is involved, determine its antibiotic sensitivity and medicate feed for 7 to 10 days. Assess the results of strategic medication.
- ❒ Inject traumatised pigs with long-acting preparations of penicillin or OTC or amoxycillin. Remove traumatised pigs from the pen to straw based accommodation.
- ❒ Increasing the salt level in the diet to 0.9% can often produce an improvement. Make sure there is an adequate and continual supply of water available.
- ❒ Spray pigs with a 1% skin antiseptic, such as savlon when ever housing is changed and continue this daily for two days.
- ❒ Spraying with a heavy industrial scent will help to reduce fighting when pigs are mixed.

Yersina Infection

(Chapter 9 pp 344)

Two species of this bacterium occur in the pig's intestine, *Y. pseudotuberculosis* and *Y. enterocolitica*. They normally cause no disease but have been associated, with minor problems in weaned pigs.

Symptoms

- ☞ *Y. enterocolitica* causes inflammation of the small and large intestines with diarrhoea and
- ☞ *Y. pseudotuberculosis* causes small tiny abscesses throughout the carcass.

Causes / Contributing factors

- ◆ This is a faeces spread disease.

Diagnosis

The main significance of the organisms is cross reactions that occur when blood tests are carried out for brucellosis. Pigs carrying the organism are likely to react positively. If this is the case it is necessary to determine the point in the rearing system when exposure takes place and break the cycle by management control.

Yersinia are easily grown in the laboratory.

Treatment

- ❒ All-in, all-out procedures with washing and disinfection will reduce infection rates.
- ❒ There is no effective treatment although antibiotics could reduce the excretion rate.

4

Managing and Treating the Sick Pig

SECTION 4

MANAGING AND TREATING THE SICK PIG

Managing and treating the sick pig

Once a sick pig has been recognised the following sequence of events is suggested:

- Identify the animal by spray or tag.
- Carefully examine the pig and its environment.
- What do you think is wrong with it? (If in doubt seek veterinary advice).
- Take the rectal temperature.
- Is it necessary to treat the condition?
- What drug has been recommended for treatment by the veterinarian?
- What nursing/welfare provisions are there?
- Should the pig be left in the pen?
- What method of drug administration should be used?
- What dose level should be given and how often should the drug be given?
- Determine method of administration, the site of injection, syringe and needle type.
- Assess the response daily.
- Normal temperature 38.6ºC to 39.5ºC (101.5 to 102.5ºF).
- Respiratory rate at 20ºC (70ºF) 25-30 per minute.

Action Points

The following points should be considered when treating the sick pig.

- Should the pig be moved immediately to a hospital pen?
- Provide a warm draught free environment.
- Are there adequate suitable pens available, easily accessible with good light?
- Can the pig access feed and water easily?

- Can you provide good nursing, good nutrition, correct medicines?
- Record all treatments.
- Will the pig be assessed twice daily?

Hospital pen requirements

- Your farm should have hospital pens.
- The floor should be solid and well drained.
- It should be deep bedded on straw, shavings or other suitable material.
- It should be well lit so that examinations are easily carried out.
- There should be easy access to food and water, preferably by a water bowl and ad lib feeder.
- One person on the farm should be appointed responsible for all sick pigs.
- There should be a maximum of six pigs per pen with a floor area of up to 1m^2 per pig for pigs up to 100kg and 3m^2 per sow.
- Adequate temperatures must be maintained in these pens and invariably this will involve either the provision of extra heating or the siting of the pens in a very warm building. To achieve this in weaners and the young growing pigs, it is necessary to provide an insulated micro-environment within the building, consisting of an insulated floor, walls and roof with an infra-red bulb or alternative heat source controlled by a thermostat. Pigs will respond much more quickly if they are in a warm, well bedded environment. On one farm regularly visited by the author all ill pigs, no matter how mild, are always moved into a series of 30 small hospital pens. The owner often relates how many of these pigs reach slaughter weight days ahead of their healthy contemporaries. There is a lesson here.

Destroying a pig

There should be facilities on the farm for humane destruction of all ages of pigs. *(See chapter 15: Slaughter).*

The design of the hospital pen

The hospital pen should be the most comfortable warm area on the farm with easy access to feed and water because the environmental requirements of the sick pig are exacting. For example the newly weaned pig affected with malabsorption will have lost most of its body fat and could require an effective temperature of 30ºC (95ºF). Hospital pens should cater for three groups of pigs, those in the immediate post-weaned period, those in the growing and finishing period and sows. In the weaning and the growing period there should be two types, one to handle the acutely ill pigs and the second to hold the recovered pigs.

This is similar to the straw based weaner accommodation *(Chapter 3 pp 98)* only smaller. It consists of an inner well heated chamber with strip curtains separated from a cooler outer section. In some designs the floor is heated as well and this provides an excellent environment. The complete pen is deep bedded with suitable materials such as straw or shavings.

Managing the sick sow

Condition	**Action**
Prolapse of the uterus.	Destroy immediately.
Prolapse of the vagina.	Replace and retain by suture.
Prolapse of the rectum.	Replace suture and casualty slaughter.
Rectal stricture.	Destroy as soon as noticed.
Open wounds.	Treat, if severe destroy.
Cuts and wounds - Mild - Severe	Treat sell when healed. Destroy.
Shoulder sores and ulcerated hocks.	Treat and move to a bedded area. Then sell when healed.
Lameness: - Off back legs. - Acutely lame.	 Destroy. Treat and assess.

Condition	Action
- Severely swollen infected .joints. - Not severe - Lame, no obvious cause but weight on all legs. - No obvious wounds and no temperature	Treat and assess or destroy. Treat and assess. Casualty slaughter or treat, if severe destroy. Treat.
Emaciated condition - Score 1	 Destroy.
Dystocia (Difficult farrowing)	Treat then review and retain only if sow expels pigs and recovers. N.B. If live pigs are present consider on-farm hysterectomy or destroy. N.B. Never send a sow with retained piglets for slaughter; in almost all countries it will be condemned.

Managing sick, growing and finishing pigs

Condition	Action
Lameness: - Totally off the back legs. - Acutely lame with swollen infected joints. - Severe. - Lame with no obvious cause, no open wounds and no temperature.	 Destroy. Treat and assess. Destroy. Casualty slaughter or treat .

Condition	Action
Severely damaged claw Recently broken legs. Severe sprains and dislocations.	Casualty slaughter or treat Destroy or casualty slaughter on the farm. Treat and assess.
Injuries: -Tail bitten. -Tail swollen, abscessed . -Tail treated / recovered. -Fresh wound. -Swelling without open wound. -Severe traumatic injuries. e.g. recent open wound. -Ear bitten, flank bitten other recent wounds. -Open Sores. -Severe open sores.	 Treat. Destroy. Sell. Consider immediate casualty slaughter. Treat. Destroy or casualty slaughter if fit to travel or treat. Treat move to hospital pen. It is essential that these cases are isolated immediately and during treatment. Move to deep bedding. Treat and assess. Slaughter when healed. Destroy.
Rectal prolapse. **Severe rectal prolapse.**	Replace and suture then sell for normal slaughter ASAP. Replace then immediately slaughter or destroy.
Ruptures: -Small . -Large but >120mm diameter. -Large with ulcerated skin.	 Sell for normal slaughter. Sell for normal slaughter at lowest possible weight. Casualty transport conditions should apply. Destroy - unfit to travel move to straw pen. Sell as normal

Condition	Action
(Cont.)	pig when recovered or casual ty slaughter if skin lesions still present at slaughter weight.
Runts and ailing pigs -Mild. -Severe.	 Treat. Destroy.
Haematoma	Check with needle if blood or abscess. Leave for 7 days and assess / lance.
Middle ear infection. -Can walk unaided.	Casualty slaughter. Treat and assess in 14 days.
Poor condition.	Assess problem. Seek veterinary advice. At least body score 2.5 for slaughter.

If you are sending a casualty pig for slaughter consider the following:

- Is it fit to travel?
- Can it stand unaided?
- Will the condition affect its suitability for consumption?
- Is suitable transport and bedding available?
- Can it be loaded without affecting its welfare?
- Can it travel the distance to the slaughter point?

Index

J

L

M

N

O

P

R

S

T

U

W

Z